Praise for *The Best Things You Can Eat*

"Kudos to David Grotto! *The Best Things You Can Eat* is well org____ ___ loaded with food as medicine pearls. Your blueprint to good health is provided in this gem of a book."

> —Gerard E. Mullin MD, author of
> *The Inside Tract: Your Good Gut Guide to Great Digestive Health*

"Dave Grotto does it again! A master at making good nutrition easy to understand with a healthy serving of great foods and lots of fun."

> —Carolyn O'Neil, MS, RD, coauthor of
> *The Dish on Eating Healthy and Being Fabulous!*

Praise for *101 Foods That Could Save Your Life:*

"An encyclopedia of foods with lifesaving benefits."

> —*Chicago Tribune*

"For the millions of Americans tired of hearing about 'what not to eat,' this book is a refreshing and enlightening guide to improving your health by adding delicious foods to your diet. Dave's simple explanations for why these foods are potential 'life savers' makes the book enjoyable to read, and the recipes bring the science to life on your plate."

> —Cynthia Sass, MPH, RD, Nutrition Director, *Prevention Magazine*

"Dave Grotto has written a book that is as fun and fascinating as it is practical. I heartily recommend *101 Foods That Could Save Your Life* as a marvelous resource for anyone who cares about their health and loves food."

> —David Katz, MD, Yale University School of Medicine
> and author of *The Flavor-Full Diet*

"*101 Foods That Could Save Your Life* is a great book to have on the shelf."

> —Brian Wansink, PhD, Cornell University Food and
> Brand Lab and author of *Mindless Eating*

"As a dietitian and food lover, I'd say this book should be opened in every kitchen."

> —Thomas Aycob, EdD, RD, Department of Pediatrics,
> Albert Einstein College of Medicine

Praise for *101 Optimal Life Foods:*

"You are holding a powerful book in your hands. David Grotto is one of the best authorities on health and nutrition in the United States today, and he has written a groundbreaking guide for you to live your ultimate, optimal life."
— Montel Williams

"This book gives you 'food for thought' about ways to use food to aide digestion, decrease inflammation and even improve your mood. Dave Grotto's simple nutritional solutions for common health conditions can easily become a part of your overall wellness routine."
— Robert Kushner, M.D., Clinical Director of the
   Northwestern Comprehensive Center on Obesity
   and author of *The Personality Type Diet*

" . . . Bonus for mid-life women: A great outline of what foods keep your skin looking youthful . . . Favorite part: The comprehensive index; find exactly what you're looking for in seconds! . . . "
— *More* magazine

"The world needs more dietitians like David—he loves food and nutrition. Your copy of *101 Optimal Life Foods* can be your best medicine."
— John La Puma, MD, director, Santa Barbara Institute
   for Medical Nutrition and Healthy Weight, and co-author
   of ChefMD's *Big Book of Culinary Medicine* and *The Real Age Diet*

the
best
things
you can
eat

For Everything from Aches to Zzzz, the Definitive Guide to the Nutrition-Packed Foods That Energize, Heal, and Help You Look Great

DAVID GROTTO, RD, LDN

Da Capo
LIFE
LONG

A Member of the Perseus Books Group

Designed by Trish Wilkinson
Set in 11 point Minion Pro by the Perseus Books Group

Library of Congress Cataloging-in-Publication Data

Grotto, David W.
The best things you can eat : for everything from aches to zzzz, the definitive guide to the nutrition-packed foods that energize, heal, and help you look great / David Grotto, RD, LDN.—First Da Capo Press edition.
    pages cm
    Includes bibliographical references and index.
    ISBN 978-0-7382-1596-9 (pbk.)—ISBN 978-0-7382-1597-6 (e-book)
1. Nutrition—Popular works.   2. Diet therapy—Popular works.   I. Title.
RA784.G763 2012
613.2—dc23
                                                                                2012035381

Published by Da Capo Press
A Member of the Perseus Books Group
www.dacapopress.com

Da Capo Press books are available at special discounts for bulk purchases in the U.S. by corporations, institutions, and other organizations. For more information, please contact the Special Markets Department at the Perseus Books Group, 2300 Chestnut Street, Suite 200, Philadelphia, PA, 19103, or call (800) 810-4145, ext. 5000, or e-mail special.markets@perseusbooks.com.

10 9 8 7 6 5 4 3 2 1

To my father and to my second mom, Sandy
Thank you for always being there!

Contents

CHAPTER 3: CHEWING THE FATS, FIBER,
           AND PHYTOSTEROLS   113

SECTION 2: BEST FOODS FOR
           WHATEVER AILS YOU

CHAPTER 4: DIGEST THIS!   141

CHAPTER 5: HEARTY FOODS   155

Acknowledgments

I am eternally grateful to all mentioned here for their help, guidance, and support.

First, I wish to thank my amazing wife, Sharon, and our three lovely daughters, Chloe, Katie, and Madison, for their extreme patience during this process. I know what a sacrifice all of you made to allow me to complete this—I love you all so very, very much!

Thanks to my research assistants Kirsten Bohrnell; Erin Dubich, MS, RD; Brian Glasser Mayrsohn; Cristian Mendoza; and Sheila Seybolt, who helped make the book come to life.

To my book advisers Lisa Young, PhD, RD; Annette Maggi, MS, RD, LD, FADA; and Roberta Duyff, MS, RD, FADA, CFCS. I appreciate your guidance on how this information should be best presented.

To my expert contributors Nancy Clark, MS, RD, CSSD; Jan Dowell, MS, MHS, RD, CSSD; Janet Brill, PhD, RD, LDN; Toby Smithson, RD, LDN; Karen Collins MS, RD, CDN; and Toby Amidor, MS, RD. Thank you for so generously sharing your wisdom!

Special thanks to Roseann Rust, RD; Christine Gerbstadt, MD, RD; Elizabeth Ward, MS, RD; Wendy Jo Peterson, MS, RD, CSSD; Joanne Lichten, PhD, RD; the Academy of Nutrition and Dietetics; Catherine Arnold, MS, EdD, RD, LDN, and the rest of the department of nutrition staff at Benedictine University; Bob True; Kirsten Straughan, MS, RD, LDN, and the staff of the Department of Nutrition Science at the University of Illinois–Chicago; my publicist, Jenna Gilligan; editor Renée Sedliar;

and everyone else involved in making this book come to life at Da Capo Lifelong Books; my literary agent, Rick Broadhead, and my speaking/ spokesperson agent, Beth Shepard.

To all of my friends, colleagues, and business associates for always supporting me and my work, I thank you from the bottom of my heart.

Foreword
By Lisa Lillien, a.k.a. "Hungry Girl"

For those of you who don't know me, I am better known as *Hungry Girl*, which is the name of my free daily email service dispensing tips, tricks, food finds, recipes and information about weight loss, dieting, making smarter food choices, and in general navigating eating in the real world. In addition to daily emails, I appear regularly on TV in my own show on Food Network & Cooking Channel and have a series of Hungry Girl books. I am also a TREMENDOUS fan of David Grotto. When I introduce myself, I often say, "I'm not a nutritionist, I'm just hungry." But when I need the advice and expertise of a top Registered Dietitian, I know where to go.

I first met Dave at an airport in Frankfurt, on the way to Italy for a food conference of sorts. That actually sounds a lot more glamorous than it was, but the meeting was quite memorable. Within minutes of being introduced to Dave, he was photographing our shoes side by side because he was amused at the size difference of our feet. Yes, Dave is easily entertained . . . (and, as an aside, he does have enormous feet). I knew instantly that Dave and I would be friends. Good friends. He is warm and funny, genuine and entertaining, and one of the smartest, most knowledgeable people I have ever met. That combination of attributes also makes him unique in his field. Too often information about health and dieting and nutrition is presented in a way that is either too convoluted, too difficult to digest (a LITTLE pun intended) or—if I am being honest—just too darn boring. Dave manages to always deliver his messages with humor and light-heartedness while always maintaining authority.

Shortly after I met Dave, a dear, lifelong friend of mine was diagnosed with adult onset diabetes. My friend didn't want to start taking pills—he wanted to combat the disease by losing weight and through better nutrition. When my friend asked me for help and advice, my first call was to Dave. He flew to Los Angeles and gave my friend a crash course in nutrition, took him grocery shopping, and made him feel better by showing him all the good things he *could* eat (as opposed to just creating a "You Can't Have This Anymore" list). Six months later, it was time for a new blood test. My friend and his doctor were shocked and thrilled by the amazing, positive results—just from eating the proper foods and losing weight. I credit Dave, along with the determination of my friend, with this great achievement.

This book is a fantastic example of Dave's amazing work. It is a lot like Dave himself. It is a book that cares, that entertains, that informs, and yet is totally relatable. We've all been told at one time or another that we needed to eat more of a certain mineral or vitamin—that we have some sort of health issue that could benefit from changing our diets. . . . Then, we often scour the Internet Googling everything possible and wind up confused, being hit with too much information and mixed messages at every turn. This book deciphers the clutter. Dave has done so much of the hard work for us and has broken it down into lovely little (dare I say!) portion-controlled bites. . . . Even those with the shortest attention spans will be able to benefit from Dave's no-nonsense approach and breezy writing style.

I know Dave, and if he could, he absolutely would personally go to each and every home and help nutritionally guide every single one of you. This book is the next best thing to making that happen.

Lisa "Hungry Girl" Lillien

Introduction

Americans have a love affair with lists. Whether it's the annual *Forbes* list of the world's richest people, *Consumer Reports'* list of the safest family vehicles, the U.S. Social Security Administration's yearly and much-anticipated release of the top baby names in the United States, or a random blogger's list of his favorite songs of the year, we love poring over rankings. They're a constant presence in newspapers, magazines, and press releases, and on talk shows (think David Letterman's daily Top Ten List) and a favorite source of content in the blogosphere, where they spread virally through e-mail and social media, providing great fodder for cocktail parties, family dinners, and even spirited arguments. The enduring popularity of lists is driven by our insatiable curiosity to know what's on them. Who wouldn't want to have a peek at a list of the "1001 Places to See Before You Die"?

Food lists are no different. When the *New York Times* ran a list of the "11 Best Foods You Aren't Eating" in 2008, intrigued readers descended on the *Times'* website en masse, making the article one of the paper's most viewed stories of all of 2009. When U.S. researchers revealed that a diet high in beta-carotene can help prolong your life, lists of beta-carotene-rich foods started popping up in articles reporting the new findings. But while these lists are helpful, they can also be overwhelming. Dietitians (like me) and medical experts are constantly bombarding us with lists of important foods, from the best sources of fiber to the best foods to eat before a workout. Keeping all of these lists clear in your head requires a spreadsheet.

The Best Things You Can Eat is the first-ever book devoted to food rankings, drawing on the latest research on food and nutrition to provide you with an irresistible compendium of food knowledge—an authoritative, informative, and enlightening go-to resource that pits one food against another and reveals the most beneficial foods in a variety of categories. If you've always wondered what food is highest in vitamin C or which foods you should rely on when you've got an upset stomach, *The Best Things You Can Eat* has the answers, and even a few surprises.

The Best Things You Can Eat is organized into three main sections: "The Vital Nutrients," which contain chapters on vitamins, minerals, fats, fibers, and phytosterols; "Best Foods for Whatever Ails You," which features information on digestion, heart health, blood glucose, oral health, and what's best for inside and out; and "Best in Show," which showcases food superstars and answers the question, "Who reigns supreme?" in categories of grains, dairy, produce, nuts, protein, and snacks, and on the best foods for working out, memory, and sleep. All in all, you'll find three sections, ten chapters, and sixty lists.

Each list is content rich, packed with intriguing facts and statistics, the latest research findings, and helpful information for healthier living. Features for each list include:

Sneak-a-peek: I'm not going to make you wait to find out how the movie ends. Turn to the beginning of each list and *bam* . . . there it is! Here's your list of top foods in each category, with their respective common serving size and exactly how much of the featured nutrient is contained within a serving.

The serving sizes featured in the lists is directly from the MyPlate.gov recommendations. They may differ from serving sizes that you see on packages, in other books, or on websites, but these are the latest and greatest recommendations modeled after the 2010 Dietary Guidelines for Americans. It also made sense to compare foods this way for establishing rankings. Other lists use a standard of 100 grams, presumably as the fairest way to make comparisons. However, if the food is light in weight, you may get an artificially high number, as in the case of ready-to-eat cereal. Let's say we wanted to compare the iron content of commonly eaten breakfast cereals, based on that 100-gram comparison. That amount would translate to about 2 cups of raisin bran and about 7 cups of puffed rice! See what I mean? Far more reasonably, the MyPlate guidelines call 1¼ cups of puffed cereal one serving; and for raisin bran, 1 cup is considered a serving. So, no worries— only common serving sizes will be featured here.

Honorable mentions: Don't you want to know which foods were at least in the running for the top spots in the list? What if you don't care much for some of the foods that made it to the Top 7? Maybe number 8 or 9 will do just fine for you. No worries—I've got you covered.

Best food groups: A theme may run throughout the list that you are interested in. For example, high-potassium foods generally fall within the fruits, vegetables, and low-fat dairy categories for foods.

What is this nutrient/condition and why is it so important? This section gives a basic overview of the nutrient or the health challenge. Deficiencies are noted and health conditions that may develop as a result of the deficiencies are addressed.

Did you know? These are great factoids, tidbits, or fascinating scientific findings about the nutrient, food, or health condition that is being featured.

How much is enough? This section takes all the guesswork out of what's recommended for your good health, whether it's an amount of a certain nutrient, or how many servings of fruit should you eat each day, sorted by age and gender.

Too much! When it comes to nutrients, more is not always better. More can be potentially dangerous if it exceeds an established upper level. This is generally more of an issue with dietary supplements than it is with overdoing a nutrient from food alone.

Supplement it? Are dietary supplements available that might help bridge the gap? What form do they come in? This section provides basic information and recommendations for supplements, but I recommend that you should always seek the advice of a registered dietitian or other qualified health professional when it comes to determining what supplement is right for you!

For each individual food featured in a list, you will find the excellent and good sources of nutrients the food or beverage supplies and study-based benefits the food offers, plus interesting information about the food itself, such as country of origin, varieties, and food lore.

Shocker food! This is the *"Whoa . . . I wasn't expecting that"* kind of a food. Some shockers include choices that are not the healthiest foods in the world, though they might be high in the featured nutrient. Case in point—chocolate! I think you will be surprised at how often chocolate appears throughout the book—I don't know about you, but I'm really happy about that! The cocoa powder in chocolate is amazingly healthy, but scarfing down a bunch of candy bars at one sitting wouldn't be. As with a good many things, moderation is the key!

A BIT ABOUT THE RANKING SYSTEM

I turned to the latest and greatest permutation of the USDA database number 24 as the authoritative guide for determining which foods reigned supreme for each of the thirty-three lists of vital nutrients. When I first began my research, I thought this section would be pretty easy to put together, as I assumed the USDA had already done the legwork and ranked foods in some sort of logical fashion. I had experience with lists of nutrient-rich foods found in other diet and nutrition books, and on the Internet, which were derived from the same database used for this book. So I thought that the only advantage of having a book like mine would be to have all of the lists together in a handy-dandy reference guide. But then I noticed something odd when I started putting together my first list on potassium. The number one highest potassium food featured on the USDA number 24 reference list was 1 cup of tomato paste! Huh? I thought, "Who sucks down a cup of tomato paste?" Maybe it was a glitch. I hurriedly skimmed to the second food on the list, only to find an equally useless recommendation for

¾ cup of frozen orange juice concentrate! Double huh?! "What do you do with frozen orange juice concentrate besides reconstitute it? I could see already that this was *not* a level playing field for the health professional or consumer.

I also observed that the USDA database included more than just foods in their original form—it also included man-made and fortified foods. For example, the number one source on the USDA list for choline was a slice of cake! (By the way, that's my "Shocker Food" for choline—I'm such a spoiler!) But seriously, what do you do with that information? So I realized I had my work cut out for me. I decided to filter the lists to contain only unfortified foods in realistic serving sizes and realistic forms of preparation (for example, cooked—not raw—liver), based on the USDA MyPlate guidelines. All I can tell you right now, because I do want you to read the rest of the book, is that this is *not* going to be your run-of-the-mill book of food lists.

I have nothing against fortification. In fact, fortifying breakfast cereals with folic acid, for one example, has had a huge positive impact on public health by seriously reducing the number of birth defects caused by folate deficiency. However, as a registered dietitian and all around healthy food guy, I'm on a mission to get my patients and readers to include more whole foods into their diet and celebrate them for their natural, unadulterated goodness. So I decided to pit foods mano a mano—standing on their own merits. Fortified foods may get an "honorable mention" in the lists but are not included in the rankings.

PERSPECTIVE

Why write such a book? Is this compendium just for those list junkies out there who crave to be the first among their friends to know who the real food winners and losers are? Well, if this describes you, get ready for some disappointment. Let me be clear. There is no such thing as a "loser" in these lists. What separates first place from first runner-up in the first thirty-three lists is a bit of subjectivity amid the objectivity of the hard numbers. As I discovered during the research process, such factors as soil condition, growing season, time of harvest, and how long foods are stored can all affect the nutrient content of foods. Also, first place and first runner-up may be separated by as little as a tenth or even a hundredth of a milligram. I also chose to feature seven top foods of each category just to give you some choice. What if beef liver comes up as the number one source of vitamin B$_{12}$ but you *hate* liver? Wouldn't you be happy to know that a 3-ounce piece of salmon would more than meet your daily needs for this nutrient? Well, of course if you hate salmon, too, you still have five more foods, plus the honorable mentions. When you come to the "Best Fruits" and the "Best Vegetables" lists, you will find that they are a bit more robust than the other "Best" lists—in fact, there are twenty top foods in those lists, to be exact. Reason? It truly is impossible to narrow down produce lists to a top three or five, due to their extensive nutrient content of vitamins, minerals, and phytochemicals.

My hopes are that this book will inspire you to eat healthier . . . not only because you will discover that a particular food is a superior source of a nutrient that you feel that you need more of, but also because the science supporting the health benefit of eating that food is so compelling that it becomes part of your dietary arsenal. So don't feel bad if you don't like a food that may be ranked first—more important, don't get so caught up in the numbers that it interferes with you eating other healthy options.

FULL DISCLOSURE

It is important for you to know that besides being an author and a clinician in private practice, I also do paid spokesperson work for commodities and brands that are in line with my nutrition philosophy. It is also important for you to know that no one has paid directly or indirectly for placement in this book. Foods sank or swam based on their own natural talents and I let science be the judge.

Always seek the guidance of a qualified health professional when taking dietary supplements.

Abbreviations Used in This Book	
Abbreviation	**Meaning**
AI	**Adequate intake** is a recommended average daily nutrient intake level, based on mean intake levels by a group (or groups) of apparently healthy people that are assumed to be adequate.
DRIs	**Dietary reference intakes** refers to a set of nutrient-based reference values based on the estimated average requirement (EAR), the recommended dietary allowance (RDA), the adequate intake (AI), and the tolerable upper intake level (UL), which can be used for planning and assessing diets. The DRIs replaced the recommended dietary allowances, which have been published since 1941 by the National Academy of Sciences and are intended to be applied to a healthy population.
DV	**Daily value** includes two sets of reference values for reporting nutrients in nutrition labeling: daily reference values (DRVs) and reference daily intakes (RDIs). DRVs are provided for total fat, saturated fat, cholesterol, total carbohydrate, dietary fiber, sodium, potassium, and protein; while RDIs provide for vitamins and minerals and for protein for children less than four years of age and for pregnant and lactating women. To limit confusion, nutrition labels on packaging use the single term *daily value* (DV) to represent both RDIs and DRVs, which are listed as a percentage of a specific nutrient that a serving of food or beverage supplies.
g	**Gram** is a metric unit of weight measurement equal to 15.432 grains, or one-thousandth of a kilogram.
IU	**International unit** is an internationally agreed-upon unit of measure defined by the International Conference for Unification of Formulae, which quantifies the activity or biological effect of substances such as fat-soluble vitamins (A, D, E, and K), enzymes, and drugs.
mg	**Milligram** is a metric unit of weight measurement equal to one-thousandth of a gram.
mcg	**Microgram** is a metric unit of weight measurement equal to one-thousandth of a milligram.
RDAs	**Recommended daily allowances** are recommended daily levels of nutrients established by the Food and Nutrition Board of the National Academy of Sciences for specific gender and age classifications, for which there is scientific consensus. In 1995, The RDA was replaced with DRI to address the needs of groups as well as individuals.
UL	**Tolerable upper intake level** is the highest level of daily nutrient intake that is likely not to pose risk of adverse health effects to most individuals. ULs could not be established for vitamin K, thiamine, riboflavin, vitamin B_{12}, pantothenic acid, biotin, and carotenoids. In the absence of a UL, precaution is suggested for not consuming levels above recommended intakes.

Section 1
THE VITAL NUTRIENTS

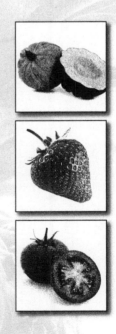

CHAPTER 1
The Vita-man Can

TOP 7 SOURCES OF VITAMIN A

SNEAK-A-PEEK: RANKINGS AT A GLANCE

Ranking	Food	Serving	Amount (IU)
First Place	Liver (cooked)	3 ounces	9,416–81,600 (see page 5)
First Runner-Up	Carrot juice (canned) Carrots (cooked)	1 cup 1 cup	45,133 26,571
Second Runner-Up	Pumpkin (canned)	1 cup	38,129
Fourth	Sweet potatoes (cooked)	1 medium	28,058
Fifth	Spinach (cooked)	1 cup	22,916
Sixth	Collard greens (cooked)	1 cup	19,538
Seventh	Kale (cooked)	1 cup	19,115

SOURCE: USDA National Nutrient Database for Standard Reference, Release 24

Honorable mentions: Beets, turnip and mustard greens, winter squash, dandelion roots (A 3½-ounce serving provides 14,000 IU, but don't eat any sprayed with weed killer!)

Best food groups: Meat (especially liver), orange and green vegetables, fortified foods

What is vitamin A and why is it so important? Vitamin A refers to a group of nutrients called retinoids that support healthy vision, skin, mucous membranes, bone growth, reproduction, and cell growth and maintenance.

3

Vitamin A is stored mainly in the liver so, not surprisingly, the liver is a good source.

Did you know? Two forms of vitamin A are found in the diet: preformed, which comes from animal sources, and provitamin A (carotenoids), which comes from plant sources. Of the 563 identified carotenoids found mainly in orange, yellow, and red fruits and vegetables, fewer than 10 percent can be made into vitamin A in the body. Night blindness is one of the earliest symptoms of vitamin A deficiency. Long-term deficiency is a leading cause of preventable blindness in children. Vitamin A deficiency can also cause increased susceptibility to infections.

HOW MUCH IS ENOUGH?

The DV for vitamin A is 5,000 IU, based on a 2,000-calorie diet.

Dietary Reference Intakes (DRIs) for Vitamin A

Age (years)	Children (mcg/day*)	Males (mcg/day)	Females (mcg/day)	Pregnancy (mcg/day)	Lactation (mcg/day)
1–3	300 (1,000 IU)				
4–8	400 (1,320 IU)				
9–13	600 (2,000 IU)				
14–18		900 (3,000 IU)	700 2,310 IU)	750 (2,500 IU)	1,200 (4,000 IU)
19+		900 (3,000 IU)	700 (2,310 IU)	770 (2,565 IU)	1,300 (4,300 IU)

*RDAs for vitamin A are given as mcg of retinol activity equivalents (RAE) to account for the different bioactivities of retinol and provitamin A carotenoids.
SOURCE: Food and Nutrition Board, Institutes of Medicine, National Academies

Too much! Excess vitamin A from animal sources can be toxic but not when it comes from plant sources, therefore there isn't a UL for beta-carotene or other provitamin A carotenoids. Beta-carotene can cause your skin to turn orange if consumed in excess. This is a harmless and reversible condition called carotenemia. Excessive retinol form of vitamin A (from animal sources), also known as hypervitaminosis A, can lead to birth defects, liver abnormalities, osteoporosis, and even death. In reality, the majority of hypervitaminosis A cases that occur are supplement, not diet, related.

Supplement it? Beta-carotene, along with other carotenoids and the retinoid form of vitamin A, are available in capsule, tablet, and liquid form. *Caution:* High-dose vitamin A in supplement form has been linked to toxicity.

First Place: Liver

Here's how they rank:

1. Moose	3 ounces braised	81,600 IU
2. Turkey	3 ounces cooked	64,033 IU
3. Veal	3 ounces braised	59,979 IU
4. Goose	3 ounces cooked	34,218 IU
5. Beef	3 ounces fried	22,175 IU
6. Lamb	3 ounces braised	22,203 IU
7. Pork	3 ounces cooked	15,297 IU
8. Chicken	3 ounces fried	12,228 IU

Liver, such as calf's liver, is one of the most nutrient-dense foods on earth. It is an excellent source of choline, copper, folate, iron, niacin, phosphorus, protein, vitamin B_{12}, and zinc, and a good source of pantothenic acid and selenium. Because animal liver has a high concentration of the most absorbable form of vitamin A, retinol, it is not advisable to eat it

Shocker Food!

Did you know that 3 ounces of polar bear liver delivers nearly 3 million IU of vitamin A? This dose is so strong that it could kill you! Even in Eskimo culture, eating polar bear liver is forbidden!

every day, especially if pregnant. Liver is fairly low in fat, but unfortunately, it is high in cholesterol, so it is advisable to limit your intake to no more than a few times per week.

First Runner-Up: Carrot Juice and Carrots

Carrot juice is an excellent source of alpha- and beta-carotene, and a good source of lutein and zeaxanthin, which are yellow pigments found concentrated in the retina of the eye. In fact, canned carrot juice contains four times more beta-carotene and five times more alpha-carotene than raw carrots. Cooking or juicing carrots helps break down their cell walls, which in turn increases the bioavailability (ability to absorb) of the carrots' beta-carotene from 5 to 90 percent! Also, a cup of carrot juice has nearly 700 milligrams of potassium, more than any other fruit or vegetable juice. Lutein and zeaxanthin, also found in unjuiced carrots, may help fight macular degeneration by blocking the absorption of blue light that causes damage to the photoreceptor cell layer.

Second Runner-Up: Pumpkin

Pumpkin (and other deep yellow winter squashes) is an excellent source of fiber, vitamin A—specifically alpha- and beta-carotene, and a good source of antioxidants. Pumpkin also contains many other nutrients, including alkaloids; flavonoids; and linoleic, oleic, and palmitic acid, which may benefit in fighting diabetes and cancer due to their antioxidant and anti-inflammatory properties.

Fourth: Sweet Potatoes

Sweet potatoes and yams look very similar, but botanically speaking, they are not even cousins. Because of the ongoing confusion among consumers, the USDA still requires that "yams" also be labeled as sweet potatoes. A large baked sweet potato is an excellent source of fiber and vitamins A, B_6, and C. It is a good source of iron, magnesium, niacin, phosphorus, potassium, riboflavin, and thiamine. Sweet potatoes may benefit diabetics in two ways: A small study showed that including sweet potatoes in diets fed to type 2 diabetics had beneficial effects on glucose control and HbA1c (a marker of long-term glucose control), along with improved insulin sensitivity. Sweet potato was also shown to decrease fibrinogen, a substance that contributes to plaque in the arteries (so they are good for heart health, too!).

Fifth: Spinach

Cooked and drained spinach is an excellent source of calcium, folate, iron, magnesium, riboflavin, and vitamins A, B_6, C, E, and K. It is a good source of fiber, phosphorus, potassium, thiamine, and zinc. Spinach has been found to have a relaxing effect on arteries, reducing the risk of heart disease as well as lowering blood pressure.

Sixth: Collard Greens

Collard greens are an excellent source of calcium, folate, manganese, and vitamins A and C. In addition, they are a good source of iron and fiber. When it comes to lowering cholesterol, cooked or steamed collards may be the way to go. One study showed that when collard greens were steamed, they possessed better bile acid–binding capacity, which helps trap cholesterol and remove it from the body, compared to raw collards.

Seventh: Kale

Chopped, cooked kale is an excellent source of vitamins A, C, and K. It is a good source of calcium, fiber, iron, phosphorus, and vitamin B_6. Kale is great juiced and terrific for your health! In fact, a study of men with high cholesterol levels who drank a little over ½ cup of kale juice everyday for 3 months saw their HDL ("good" cholesterol) and HDL to LDL ratios significantly increase by 27 and 52 percent, respectively. Their LDL ("bad" cholesterol) also was reduced.

TOP 7 SOURCES OF
THIAMINE (VITAMIN B₁)

SNEAK-A-PEEK: RANKINGS AT A GLANCE

Ranking	Food	Serving	Amount (mg)
First Place	Pork, lean (cooked)	3 ounces	0.53
First Runner-Up	Soybeans (cooked)	1 cup	0.468
Second Runner-Up	Peas (cooked)	1 cup	0.453
Fourth	Cowpeas (cooked)	1 cup	0.442
Fifth	Navy beans (cooked)	1 cup	0.431
Sixth	Black beans (cooked)	1 cup	0.42
Seventh	Lentils (cooked)	1 cup	0.335

SOURCE: USDA National Nutrient Database for Standard Reference, Release 24

Honorable mentions: Fortified cereals and bread products, oat bran, beef liver, asparagus, tahini (sesame butter), Marmite (yeast paste)

Best food groups: Pork, legumes, seeds, fortified breakfast cereals

What is thiamine and why is it so important? Thiamine, also known as vitamin B₁, is one of the B-complex nutrients which are essential in energy metabolism. Deficiencies in thiamine have been linked to beriberi, peripheral neuritis, pellagra, poor appetite, ulcerative colitis, and diarrhea. Thiamine supplementation is also used as medical therapy for diverse health conditions, such as AIDS and other immuno-compromised conditions, and alcoholism. Research has also shown promising results in the treatment of kidney damage.

HOW MUCH IS ENOUGH?

The DV for thiamine is 1.5 mg, based on a 2,000-calorie diet.

Dietary Reference Intakes (DRIs) for Vitamin B₁ (Thiamine)

Age (years)	Children (mg/day)	Males (mg/day)	Females (mg/day)	Pregnancy (mg/day)	Lactation (mg/day)
1–3	0.5				
4–8	0.6				
9–13		0.9	0.9		
14–18		1.2	1.0	1.4	1.4
19+		1.2	1.1	1.4	1.4

SOURCE: Food and Nutrition Board, Institutes of Medicine, National Academies

Too much! There is no UL for thiamine. No adverse effects have been observed with high intakes.

Supplement it? For adults with somewhat low levels of thiamine in their body (mild thiamine deficiency), the usual dose of thiamine is 5 to 30 mg daily in either a single dose or divided doses for 1 month. The typical dose for severe deficiency can be up to 300 mg per day. For reducing the risk of cataracts, a daily dietary intake of about 10 mg of thiamine is recommended. You'll find thiamine in individual supplements as well as multivitamins.

First Place: Lean Pork

Besides being an excellent source of thiamine, lean pork is an excellent source of niacin, protein, selenium, and vitamin B_{12}, and a good source of vitamin B_6. According to National Health and Nutrition Examination Survey (NHANES) data for 2003–2006, diets that included lean pork provided higher amounts of protein, selenium, thiamine, and vitamin B_6, compared to the diets of adults who did not consume lean pork.

First Runner-Up: Soybeans

Cooked soybeans are an excellent source of calcium, fiber, folate, iron, magnesium, phosphorus, potassium, riboflavin, thiamine, and vitamin K. It is a good source of niacin, vitamin C, and zinc. Soy is already an excellent source of thiamine but a German study found that the bacteria used in the fermentation process in making tempeh (a traditional Japanese fermented soybean cake) intensified the amounts of niacin, nicotinamide, thiamine, and vitamin B_{12}.

Shocker Food!

Marmite is a smoky-tasting spread made from brewer's yeast, a by-product of the brewing process. Although yeast is naturally high in B vitamins, the makers of Marmite add thiamine (and other assorted B vitamins) to their spread for an extra boost. It's a popular spread around the world but hasn't really caught on that well in the United States. It's delicious as a sandwich spread or even as a marinade ingredient.

Second Runner-Up: Green Peas

Green peas are an excellent source of not only thiamine, but the carotenoids lutein and zeaxanthin, and a good source of vitamin K, fiber, and folate. Fresh green peas are high in the plant nutrient beta-sitosterol, which helps block the absorption of cholesterol.

Fourth: Cowpeas

Cowpeas are also known as Southern peas or black-eyed peas. Cowpeas are an excellent source of calcium, fiber, thiamine, and vitamin A, and a good source of iron. Cowpeas are rich in phytic acid and a group of plant nutrients called polyphenols, which are found mainly in their hull. Removing the hull after soaking them for twelve hours is a great way to reduce phytic acid, which can interfere with calcium absorption; however, nearly 70 percent of the healthy polyphenols are stripped away by that process, too.

Fifth: Navy Beans

Navy beans are an excellent source of fiber, folate, protein, and thiamine, and a good source of iron and magnesium. Navy beans also contain saponins, a phytochemical that has been shown to have antibacterial and antifungal activity, not to mention anticancer cell growth. Navy beans are also the highest common bean source of ferulic and p-coumaric acids, antioxidants shown to protect against breast, liver, and stomach cancers. A small study showed that including navy beans in a meal busted hunger earlier and led to lower blood glucose following the meal, compared to meals that contained lentils, yellow peas, or chickpeas.

Navy beans are a variety of white bean that received their nickname because they were served so often to American naval personal during the latter part of the nineteenth century. Other navy bean varieties include the great northern, Rainy River, Robust, Michelite, and Sanilac.

Sixth: Black Beans

Black beans are an excellent source of fiber and protein. When served with rice, they make an inexpensive complete protein meal. Besides providing thiamine, black beans are also an excellent source of folate, iron, magnesium, manganese, molybdenum, and phosphorus, and a good source of potassium and zinc. A Canadian study found that black beans exhibited powerful anti-inflammatory properties, even outperforming aspirin for blocking COX-1 and COX-2, enzymes known to cause inflammation!

Seventh: Lentils

Lentils are an excellent source of fiber, folate, iron, magnesium, manganese, phosphorus, thiamine, vitamin B_6, and zinc. A study of over four hundred Iranian women found that those consuming greater amounts of lentils and other legumes in their diet had much lower concentrations of inflammatory markers in their blood.

TOP 7 SOURCES OF RIBOFLAVIN (VITAMIN B_2)

SNEAK-A-PEEK: RANKINGS AT A GLANCE

Ranking	Food	Serving	Amount (mg)
First Place	Beef liver (cooked)	3 ounces	3.0
First Runner-Up	Cottage cheese	2 cup	0.90
Second Runner-Up	Yogurt	1 cup	0.53
Fourth	Soybeans (cooked)	1 cup	0.49
Fifth	White mushrooms (cooked)	1 cup	0.47
Sixth	Milk (2%)	1 cup	0.45
Seventh	Spinach (cooked)	1 cup	0.43

SOURCE: USDA National Nutrient Database for Standard Reference, Release 24

Honorable mentions: Fortified cereals, malted milk, wheat flour, eggs, almonds

Best food groups: Meat, dairy, legumes, fortified grains

What is riboflavin and why is it so important? Riboflavin is a water-soluble nutrient that was first identified in the whey protein component of milk back in 1879 and was then named lactochrome. It is an integral nutrient in the conversion of food into energy and the elimination of drugs and toxins by the liver. It is also needed for healthy skin, digestion, and healthy blood cells. Low levels of riboflavin often occur in combination with deficiencies of other water-soluble vitamins and can also be due to malabsorption conditions, such as celiac disease, ulcerative colitis, and Crohn's disease; malignancies; and alcoholism. Symptoms of riboflavin deficiencies include: sore throat, cracks or sores on the lips and at the corners of the mouth, inflamed tongue, moist and scaly skin, and normochromic-normocytic anemia.

Riboflavin deficiency is a concern for those who exist on vegetarian diets lacking dairy products and meat. Vitamin supplementation and/or fortified foods are necessary to meet dietary needs in poorly planned vegan diets, but are usually not a problem in those that include a diverse selection of fruits and riboflavin-rich vegetables, such as spinach.

Did you know? A small cross-sectional study of ninety-eight female clinical nurses evaluated them for depression and also assessed their dietary intake of riboflavin. Researchers found that riboflavin deficiencies were more prevalent in depressed subjects.

HOW MUCH IS ENOUGH?

The DV for riboflavin is 1.7 mg, based on a 2,000-calorie diet.

Dietary Reference Intakes (DRIs) for Vitamin B$_2$ (Riboflavin)

Age (years)	Children (mg/day)	Males (mg/day)	Females (mg/day)	Pregnancy (mg/day)	Lactation (mg/day)
1–3	0.5				
4–8	0.6				
9–13		0.9	0.9		
14–18		1.3	1.0	1.4	1.4
19+		1.3	1.1	1.4	1.4

SOURCE: Food and Nutrition Board, Institutes of Medicine, National Academies

Too much! There is no UL for riboflavin. High amounts have not been found harmful in humans.

Supplement it? All multivitamins contain riboflavin. According to the *Natural Medicines Comprehensive Database,* riboflavin supplementation is effective for not only treating riboflavin deficiency, but may reduce the number of migraine headaches and may also play a role in preventing cataracts.

First Place: Beef Liver

See page 286 for the full story on beef liver's health riches. Inadequate riboflavin intake can impair the absorption of iron. The great thing about liver is that it's high in both!

Shocker Food! ───────────

A 3-ounce serving (three slices) of braunschweiger supplies 1.3 mg of riboflavin. Also known as smoked liverwurst, this sausage is an excellent source of vitamin A and a good source of iron, niacin, and selenium. See also page 290.

First Runner-Up: Cottage Cheese

Low-fat (1%) cottage cheese is an excellent source of phosphorus, riboflavin, and vitamin B_{12}, and a good source of calcium and vitamin B_6. Low-fat dairy products, such as cottage cheese, were found in a cost analysis conducted by Adam Drewnowski, PhD, to be one of the lowest-cost sources of dietary calcium and riboflavin, among other nutrients.

Second Runner-Up: Yogurt

Of all dairy products, yogurt is most concentrated in calcium, iodine, and potassium. It is also an excellent source of phosphorus, protein, riboflavin, and vitamin B_{12}. Undergoing chemotherapy for the treatment of cancer can have profound side effects, including malnutrition. Cisplatin, a chemotherapy agent, can cause damage to the kidneys and liver. A study found that groups that were treated with the combination of cisplatin and riboflavin showed reduced toxicity to those organs. Yogurt is not only rich in riboflavin, but also contains helpful friendly bacteria called probiotics that help maintain a healthy immune system.

Fourth: Soybeans

For the full health story on soybeans, see page 291. A large study found that those with higher levels of riboflavin in their blood had lower risk of colorectal cancer. This was also true of another B vitamin, folate, of which soybeans are a rich source.

Fifth: White Mushrooms

Riboflavin is an important nutrient for detoxification. Low in calories, mushrooms not only provide this vitamin, but also contain powerful antioxidants that help the riboflavin neutralize toxins and reduce free radical damage to the body. Not only are mushrooms are an excellent source of selenium and a good source of niacin and pantothenic acid, but they are the highest vegetarian source of vitamin D. White button mushrooms were shown to have anticancer effects both in cell and animal studies. Some research suggests that the conjugated linoleic acid found in white mushrooms may help fight against prostate cancer.

Sixth: Milk

Low-fat (2%) milk is an excellent source of calcium, phosphorus, and vitamins B_{12} and D. It is a good source of vitamin A and zinc. Dairy products, such as milk, contribute over 50 percent of riboflavin needs in preschool children, 35 percent in schoolchildren, 27 percent in adults, and 36 percent in the elderly.

Seventh: Spinach

Cooked and drained spinach is an excellent source of riboflavin. See page 291 for the many other nutrients in these dark leafy greens.

TOP 7 SOURCES OF NIACIN
(VITAMIN B$_3$)

SNEAK-A-PEEK: RANKINGS AT A GLANCE

Ranking	Food	Serving	Amount (mg)
First Place	Yellowfin tuna (cooked)	3 ounces	19.0
First Runner-Up	Beef liver (cooked)	3 ounces	15.0
Second Runner-Up	Chicken breast (cooked)	3 ounces	12.0
Fourth	Veal, top round (cooked)	3 ounces	9.0
Fifth	Pork loin, boneless (cooked)	3 ounces	8.5
Sixth	Sockeye salmon (cooked)	3 ounces	8.2
Seventh	Swordfish (cooked)	3 ounces	8.0

SOURCE: USDA National Nutrient Database for Standard Reference, Release 24

Honorable mentions: Sirloin beef, whole-grain wheat, buckwheat groats, mushrooms, lamb

Best food groups: Meat, fish, fortified cereals, grain products

What is niacin and why is it so important? Niacin (nicotinic acid) is a member of the B-complex family. Another form of niacin called niacinamide is needed to help make adenosine-5'-triphosphate (ATP), which provides energy to every cell in the body.

Niacin deficiencies can occur from following a low-protein diet and not taking a dietary supplement containing the vitamin. Pellagra is a disease caused by severe niacin deficiency and is often associated with the "4 Ds": dermatitis, diarrhea, dementia, and death. In the early 1900s, pellagra was commonplace in the southern United States among the poor, whose diet consisted mainly of corn. However, pellagra is relatively unknown in Mexico or among Native Americans, where corn is a staple of the diet: Because their traditional method of preparation involves soaking corn in a lime (calcium hydroxide) solution before cooking, this process releases the niacin that is bound within the grain, to be used by the body. This fact is not lost on modern food manufacturers—check out corn chips and tortillas and see whether the label lists lime as an ingredient.

HOW MUCH IS ENOUGH?

The DV for niacin is 20 mg, based on a 2,000-calorie diet.

Dietary Reference Intakes (DRIs) for Vitamin B₃ (Niacin)

Age	Children (mg/day)	Males (mg/day)	Females (mg/day)	Pregnancy (mg/day)	Lactation (mg/day)
0–6 months	2				
6–12 months	4				
1–3 years	6				
4–8 years	8				
9–13 years		12	12		
14–18 years		16	14	18	17
19+ years		16	14	18	17

SOURCE: Food and Nutrition Board, Institutes of Medicine, National Academies

Too much! The UL of 35 mg is due to the flushing (reddening) effect niacin has on the body, but much higher doses are given to treat such health conditions as elevated cholesterol. Headache, diarrhea, upset stomach, and vomiting occur in 2 to 10 percent of consumers in doses ranging from 500 to 3,000 mg per day. Toxic liver effects can occur at the 3 to 9 g per day range and can result in jaundice and elevated liver enzymes.

Did you know? Dr. Abram Hoffer, an orthomolecular psychiatrist and chemist, discovered that niacin can reduce total cholesterol and raise HDL cholesterol.

Supplement it? Niacin is used at high doses as a cholesterol-lowering agent and is sold as a prescription drug. Niacinamide does not cause flushing and can be used in higher doses than the recommended UL for niacin.

First Place: Yellowfin Tuna

Canned tuna is most likely to be yellowfin, skipjack, or albacore. In addition to being an excellent source of niacin, tuna is an excellent source of protein, selenium, and vitamin B₁₂, and a good source of pantothenic acid. A National Institute for Occupational Safety and Health study looked at the role of niacin in protecting against ionizing radiation in airplane pilots. Those pilots with the highest dietary intake of niacin-rich foods, such as tuna, accompanied with lower processed red meat intake, displayed less chromosome damage, compared to the others.

First Runner-Up: Beef Liver

For the full scoop on beef liver's healthy properties, see page 286.

Second Runner-Up: Chicken Breast

Chicken breast is an excellent source of niacin and protein, and a good source of choline, pantothenic acid, and selenium. Choose chicken breast if you can; dark meat has about half the niacin found in light meat. Skinless chicken breast is low in cholesterol, too—only 73 mg. Chicken breast is higher in the amino acid tryptophan, known for promoting relaxation and sleep, than turkey breast—which most believe is the other way around. But it might not make any difference, as tryptophan must compete with other amino acids to cross the blood-brain barrier. So the post–Thanksgiving meal snooze-fest may be due to eating too large a meal, rather than to the effects of tryptophan.

Fourth: Veal

The veal from exclusively milk-fed calves is pale pink, whereas that from grain-fed calves is darker in color. Lean veal is an excellent source of niacin and protein, and a good source of riboflavin, vitamin B_{12}, and zinc. A Spanish study found that participants who consumed either lean pork or lean veal as part of a heart-healthy diet lowered their LDL cholesterol an average of 5.5 percent.

Fifth: Pork Loin

A lean pork chop is an excellent source of niacin, protein, selenium, and vitamin B_{12}, and a good source of vitamin B_6. According to a recent NHANES study, pork accounts for 11 to 19 percent of total niacin intake in the United States.

Shocker Food! —

Animal protein by far supplies the richest source of niacin; however, 1 cup of cooked white mushrooms is an excellent source of niacin and supplies 7 mg per cup—nearly one-third of the daily value! See page 289 for the additional benefits of mushrooms.

Sixth: Sockeye Salmon

Sockeye salmon is an excellent source of niacin, protein, selenium, and vitamins B_{12} and D; and a good source of choline, omega-3 fatty acids, thiamine, and vitamin B_6. A Spanish study found that pregnant women who added two servings of salmon to their diet weekly had enhanced antioxidant defenses, compared to those women who didn't.

Seventh: Swordfish

Swordfish is an excellent source of niacin, protein, and vitamin D, and a good source of choline and vitamins B_6 and B_{12}. Swordfish are also a great source of omega-3 fatty acids. A study found that a 3.5-ounce portion of swordfish delivered over 2 g of omega-3s! Pregnant women, lactating mothers, and young children are advised not to eat swordfish because its mercury levels remain high.

TOP 7 SOURCES OF PANTOTHENIC ACID (VITAMIN B$_5$)

SNEAK-A-PEEK: RANKINGS AT A GLANCE

Ranking	Food	Serving	Amount (mg)
First Place	Beef liver (cooked)	3 ounces	5.9
First Runner-Up	Shiitake mushrooms (raw)	1 cup	5.2
Second Runner-Up	Braunschweiger	3 slices 3 ounces	2.86
Fourth	Trout (cooked)	3 ounces	1.69
Fifth	Yogurt	1 cup	1.45
Sixth	Sweet corn	1 cup	1.418
Seventh	Lobster (cooked)	3 ounces	1.417

SOURCE: USDA National Nutrient Database for Standard Reference, Release 24

Honorable mentions: Peas, chocolate milk, crab, sweet potatoes, potatoes, pork, lentils

Best food groups: Fortified cereals, meat, fish, vegetables, dairy, legumes, and eggs

What is pantothenic acid and why is it so important? Pantothenic acid is a water-soluble nutrient that belongs to the B-complex family of vitamins and is also known as vitamin B_5. Along with the other B vitamins, pantothenic acid helps in the conversion of carbohydrates from food into glucose for energy. Pantothenic acid also supports healthy hair, skin, eyes; liver health, including cholesterol production; healthy nervous and reproductive system function; red blood cell production; adrenal gland function; and healthy digestion.

Although pantothenic acid deficiencies are usually rare because of its abundance in fortified foods, deficiency symptoms can include upper respiratory infections, depression, nausea and vomiting, digestive upset, fatigue, and burning feet and hands.

Did you know? Eating a diet rich in pantothenic acid may help halt the aging of the skin! A study found that a vitamin B_5 deficiency decreased the production and health of keratinocytes, the most common type of skin cell.

HOW MUCH IS ENOUGH?

The DV for pantothenic acid is 10 mg, based on a 2,000-calorie diet.

Dietary Reference Intakes (DRIs) for Vitamin B_5 (Pantothenic Acid)

Age	Children (mg/day)	Males (mg/day)	Females (mg/day)	Pregnancy (mg/day)	Lactation (mg/day)
0–6 months	1.7				
6–12 months	1.8				
1–3 years	2				
4–8 years	3				
9–13 years		4	4		
14–18 years		5	5	6	7
19–50 years		5	5	6	7
51–70 years		5	5		
71+ years		5	5		

SOURCE: Food and Nutrition Board, Institutes of Medicine, National Academies

Too much! No UL has been created for pantothenic acid; however, large doses (10 g or more) may cause diarrhea.

Supplement it? Pantothenic acid can be found in B-complex and multivitamin formulas and as a single agent. It comes in tablet, capsule, and softgel forms mainly as calcium or sodium pantothenate, which are both equally effective. It is also available as the metabolically active form, pantethine, for which research supports its usefulness in helping to manage blood lipids.

First Place: Beef Liver

See page 286 for the full scoop on beef liver's healthy attributes. Liver provides many additional key nutrients that, working in conjunction with pantothenic acid, support reproductive health. An animal research study showed that significantly decreased testosterone and sperm motility occurred in the test group that ate a pantothenic acid–deprived diet, compared to the control group.

First Runner-Up: Shiitake Mushrooms

Shiitakes are the second most-cultivated species, following the common button mushroom. China is the world's biggest producer, with more than 1.6 million tons. Shiitake mushrooms not only have a meaty flavor, but hold their own when compared with animal proteins for pantothenic acid content! Shiitake mushrooms are an excellent source of copper and a good source of niacin, phosphorus, riboflavin, and vitamins B_6 and E. Shiitake mushrooms are also rich in beta-glucan, a plant nutrient known for reducing cholesterol and boosting immune function. In addition, in a human cell study, shiitake mushrooms caused plaque-building adhesion molecules to become dormant.

Second Runner-Up: Braunschweiger

For the full scoop on the healthy benefits of braunschweiger, see page 290, Traditionally, braunschweiger is made from pork liver, but there are beef, turkey, and even bison versions that are even leaner.

Fourth: Trout

Besides its pantothenic acid content, which research shows to reduce cholesterol, rainbow trout is an excellent source of cholesterol-lowering omega-3 fatty acids and also protein, and a good source of niacin and selenium.

Fifth: Yogurt

See page 292 for more info on the benefits of yogurt. The pantothenic acid in yogurt helps fight fatigue and convert glycogen stores in muscles into glucose for energy, which makes it especially great for athletes. Probiotics in yogurt may enhance athletic performance by optimizing immune health and maintaining a healthy gastrointestinal tract.

Sixth: Corn

Aside from its pantothenic acid content, sweet corn is also a good source of fiber, manganese, niacin, and vitamin C. The bran of corn contains the highest level of pantothenic acid, compared to the remaining components of the kernel. When it comes to dried corn bran or cornmeal, the finer it is ground, the greater the bioavailability of this vitamin and many other nutrients.

Seventh: Lobster

Besides being rich in pantothenic acid, lobster is a great lean option for protein, while also providing phosphorus and selenium. Some may think it is really high in cholesterol because it's a crustacean. However, lobster is lower in cholesterol than most other animal products. A 3-ounce serving only has about 60 mg of cholesterol, which is well below the daily recommendation of 300 mg per day.

TOP 7 SOURCES OF PYRIDOXINE (VITAMIN B$_6$)

SNEAK-A-PEEK: RANKINGS AT A GLANCE

Ranking	Food	Serving	Amount (mg)
First Place	Chickpeas (cooked)	1 cup	1.14
First Runner-Up	Yellowfin tuna (cooked)	3 ounces	0.90
Second Runner-Up	Beef liver (cooked)	3 ounces	0.873
Fourth	Pork loin, boneless (cooked)	3 ounces	0.60
Fifth	Sockeye salmon (cooked)	3 ounces	0.59
Sixth	Prune juice	1 cup	0.56
Seventh	Bananas	1 cup	0.55

SOURCE: USDA National Nutrient Database for Standard Reference, Release 24

Honorable mentions: Fortified cereal, swordfish, turkey giblets, chicken breast, plantains

Best food groups: Fish, beef liver and other organ meats, potatoes and other starchy vegetables, noncitrus fruit

What is vitamin B$_6$ and why is it so important? Vitamin B$_6$, also known as pyridoxine, is a water-soluble nutrient that is a member of the B-complex family. B$_6$ is most known for helping to convert stored energy, known as glycogen, and amino acids into glucose. B$_6$ also assists in making the brain chemicals that govern mood: the neurotransmitters serotonin, dopamine, norepinephrine, and gamma-aminobutyric acid (commonly known as GABA).

Deficiencies in B$_6$ often first manifest as confusion or depression. Other deficiency signs include mouth sores; tongue inflammation; and ulcers of the skin surrounding the mouth.

Did you know? Studies show high-dose vitamin B$_6$ supplementation may benefit some children and adults with autism.

HOW MUCH IS ENOUGH?

The DV for B_6 is 2 mg, based on a 2,000-calorie diet.

Dietary Reference Intakes (DRIs) for Vitamin B_6

Age	Children (mg/day)	Males (mg/day)	Females (mg/day)	Pregnancy (mg/day)	Lactation (mg/day)
0–6 months	0.1				
7–12 months	0.3				
1–3 years	0.5				
4–8 years	0.6				
9–13 years		1.0	1.0		
14–18 years		1.3	1.2	1.9	2.0
19–50 years		1.3	1.3	1.9	2.0
51+ years		1.7	1.5		

SOURCE: Food and Nutrition Board, Institutes of Medicine, National Academies

Too much! The UL for adults is 100 mg. Ironically, neuropathies (damaged nervous tissue) are a sign of a B_6 deficiency, but excessive amounts of this vitamin have been associated with neuropathy as well. Sensory neuropathy can occur at doses lower than 500 mg per day; however, some studies found that those who were taking up to 200 mg per day for a period up to five years did not suffer from neuropathy.

Supplement it? You can find vitamin B_6 in liquid, capsule, tablet, and chewable form, in a variety of formulas, including multivitamins, B-complex vitamins, and as a single agent. The most common form is pyridoxine hydrochloride, although a more expensive pyridoxal phosphate (PLP) form is available. Most B_6 deficiency scenarios are well addressed with vastly less expensive pyridoxine hydrochloride.

First Place: Chickpeas

For most of the B vitamins, animal proteins generally reign supreme in being the richest source. Surprisingly, chickpeas, otherwise known as garbanzos, top any other food (excepted fortified foods) in supplying the most vitamin B_6 per serving. Chickpeas are legumes that were first culti-vated in the Mediterranean region back in 3000 BC. Chickpeas are also an excellent source of copper, fiber, folate, manganese, molybdenum, and protein, and a good source of magnesium. Two small, randomized and separate studies found that diets that included chickpeas helped lower to-tal cholesterol and harmful LDL cholesterol better than the control diet.

First Runner-Up: Yellowfin Tuna

For the full scoop on the benefits of yellowfin tuna, see page 292. Vitamin B_6 is instrumental in the production of brain neurotransmitters that help boost mood and keep depression in check. In a study of 618 elderly sub-jects who were tested for depressive symptoms, there was a significant correlation with low B_6 levels in their diet. Tuna has the benefit of high B_6 levels, plus omega-3 fatty acids, which have been shown to combat depression.

Second Runner-Up: Beef Liver

For the full story on beef liver's healthy properties, see page 286. A 2004 NHANES study of over six thousand people found that many adult males who did not take B_6 supplements had compromised B_6 levels. However, re-search suggests that women of childbearing years, especially those who were taking oral contraceptives, had considerably lower levels of vitamin B_5 than did men. Beef liver provides much-needed B_6, iron, and folate, which are important nutrients for women who are not in menopause.

Fourth: Pork Loin

For the full scoop on boneless pork loin, see page 290. In a study of women over the age of fifty-five, those women who did not consume a diet rich in vitamin B_6 foods, such as pork, or take B_6 supplements were often deficient and also had elevated levels of homocysteine, an inflamma-tory marker associated with increased risk for heart disease.

Fifth: Sockeye Salmon

For more detail on sockeye salmon, see page 291. As mentioned earlier with tuna, omega-3 fatty acids, combined with vitamin B_6, can be quite helpful in fighting depression. Salmon is rich in docosahexaenoic acid (DHA), a form of omega-3s that has been well studied in its ability to protect and stimulate cognition and learning centers in the brain.

Sixth: Prune Juice

Besides being an excellent source of vitamin B_6, prunes are also a good source of vitamin A and fiber, and are loaded with polyphenols that help fight heart disease and cancer. Vitamin B_6 has mild diuretic qualities and may help in controlling hypertension. Prune juice also contains additional plant nutrients known to exert a positive effect on blood pressure and cholesterol.

Seventh: Bananas

Bananas are a good source of fiber, manganese, potassium, and vitamin C. An animal study showed that the absorption of vitamin B_6 was slightly lower from bananas than from animal products. However, bananas are still considered an excellent source of B_6.

TOP 7 SOURCES OF BIOTIN (VITAMIN B_7)

SNEAK-A-PEEK: RANKINGS AT A GLANCE

Ranking	Food	Serving	Amount (mcg)
First Place	Chicken liver (cooked)	3 ounces	158
First Runner-Up	Beef liver (cooked)	3 ounces	35.38
Second Runner-Up	Eggs (cooked)	1 large	10
Fourth	Salmon (cooked)	3 ounces	4.98
Fifth	Peanuts	1 ounce	4.91
Sixth	Pork chop (cooked)	3 ounces	3.79
Seventh	Mushrooms (canned)	1 cup	2.59

SOURCE: *Journal of Food Composition and Analysis* 17, no. 6. (December 2004), 767–76.

Honorable mentions: Cereal, chocolate, legumes, dairy, nuts, beef liver, yeast

Best food groups: Enriched cereal grains, meat, eggs, dairy

What is biotin and why is it so important? Biotin, or vitamin B_7, is a water-soluble B vitamin that was first discovered in 1927 but took nearly forty years to be fully recognized as a nutrient. Biotin is required by all organisms. It can be created by bacteria, yeasts, molds, algae, and some plants, but not humans. It is important in the maintenance of all cells in the body and supports healthy skin and hair, the nervous and digestive systems, and carbohydrate metabolism.

Deficiencies, once thought to be rare, are a concern and may present as dry, scaly skin, nausea, anorexia, dermatitis, hair loss, conjunctivitis, depression, and hallucinations.

Did you know? Biotin was once referred to as several different terms, such as coenzyme R, vitamin H, and "the anti–egg white factor." (Raw egg whites contain a biotin binding protein called avidin; however, when egg whites are cooked, avidin is destroyed.)

HOW MUCH IS ENOUGH?

The DV for biotin is 300 mcg, based on a 2,000-calorie diet.

Dietary Reference Intakes (DRIs) for Vitamin B_7 (Biotin)

Age	Children (mcg/day)	Males (mcg/day)	Females (mcg/day)	Pregnancy (mcg/day)	Lactation (mcg/day)
0–6 months	5				
6–12 months	6				
1–3 years	8				
4–8 years	12				
9–13 years		20	20		
14–18 years		25	25	30	35
19–50 years		30	30	30	35
51+ years		30	30		

SOURCE: Food and Nutrition Board, Institutes of Medicine, National Academies

Too much! Biotin is not known to be toxic. Doses up to 200,000 mcg per day for short periods of time and doses up to 5,000 mcg per day for up to two years were all reported to be well tolerated. Therefore, the Institutes of Medicine (IOM) have not established a UL for biotin.

Supplement it? High doses have been used to treat peripheral neuropathy, elevated blood glucose, insulin resistance, and elevated blood lipids. Popular use of biotin in the dietary supplement form is to treat hair loss or to make hair thicker. To date, the research to support its use for this purpose is rather weak.

First Place: Chicken Liver

No other food even comes close, including livers from other animal sources, in supplying biotin in the diet. Chicken liver is also an excellent source of choline (255 percent of DV), folate (127 percent of DV), iron, niacin, pantothenic acid, phosphorus, riboflavin, selenium (over 100 percent of DV), vitamin A, vitamin B_{12} (247 percent of DV), and zinc; and a good source of the phytochemicals lutein, lycopene, and zeaxanthin. It's even fairly low in saturated fat! If it weren't for that pesky ol' 495 mg of cholesterol per serving, chicken liver might be one the healthiest foods in the whole book! Research suggests that many pregnant women are marginally biotin deficient and that this deficiency can lead to birth defects. Certainly, taking a prenatal formula can address a biotin deficiency; however, also eating biotin-rich foods such as chicken liver provides an abundance of this and other nutrients in a fairly small portion. In addition, biotin helps in the formation of heme, which aids in iron absorption.

First Runner-Up: Beef Liver

For the healthy scoop on beef liver, see page 285. Animal research has shown that both biotin and chromium deficiencies can contribute to poor glucose management and reduced insulin sensitivity, leading to metabolic syndrome and diabetes. Beef liver is a good source of both biotin and chromium.

Second Runner-Up: Eggs

Eggs are a good source of phosphorus, protein, riboflavin, and vitamin D. Biotin is instrumental in gene expression that protects the brain. Eggs not only provide a source of biotin but also brain-friendly choline, which may help in improving cognition.

Fourth: Pink Salmon

For the lowdown on salmon's healthy properties, see page 291. Biotin controls gene expression that's critical in the regulation of blood glucose and cholesterol production. A diet that includes biotin and omega-3 fatty acid–containing foods, such as salmon, may help control lipid and blood glucose disorders.

Fifth: Peanuts

One ounce of peanuts is an excellent source of manganese and niacin, and a good source of copper, fiber, folate, magnesium, phosphorus, thiamine, vitamin E, and zinc. A human cell study found that lymphoma cancer cells that were biotin deficient were more resistant to the killing effects of the chemotherapeutic drugs doxorubicin and vinblastine. Peanuts are a nutritious snack that contains biotin as well as a host of nutrients that help bolster the nutrition status of cancer patients undergoing chemotherapy.

Sixth: Pork Chop

For more about the healthy properties of lean pork, see page 290. Lean protein, such as pork, has been shown to help control blood glucose, manage weight by increasing satiety, and also help preserve lean muscle tissue. There are seven cuts of pork that qualify as "lean" (under 10 grams of fat). The fat in lean pork is made up of mostly trans fat–free mono- and polyunsaturated fat, which fits well into a heart-healthy diet.

Seventh: Mushrooms

For more on the health benefits of mushrooms, see pages 14, 20, and 289. For the vegetarians out there or those who simply want to reduce their meat intake, mushrooms offer a real solution. A study that swapped out calorie-dense meats and substituted mushrooms found that calorie intake was significantly higher when meat meals were consumed, but the volume of food between the meat and mushroom meals were the same. The best news is that most subjects did not rate palatability, appetite, or the feeling of being full and satisfied for the mushroom meals any differently than for the meat meals.

TOP 7 SOURCES OF FOLATE
(VITAMIN B₉)

SNEAK-A-PEEK: RANKINGS AT A GLANCE

Ranking	Food	Serving	Amount (mcg)
First Place	Chicken liver (cooked)	3 ounces	491
First Runner-Up	Lentils (cooked)	1 cup	358
Second Runner-Up	Cowpeas (cooked)	1 cup	358
Fourth	Pinto beans (cooked)	1 cup	294
Fifth	Chickpeas (cooked)	1 cup	282
Sixth	Spinach (cooked)	1 cup	263
Seventh	Black beans (cooked)	1 cup	256

Source: USDA National Nutrient Database for Standard Reference, Release 24

Honorable mentions: Enriched grains, cereals

Best food groups: Enriched cereal grains, vegetables

What is folate and why is it so important? You may have seen the terms *folate* and *folic acid* used interchangeably for the same nutrient. Folate is the water-soluble B-complex nutrient as it naturally occurs in food; folic acid is the synthetically made equivalent of folate. The relationship between folate deficiency and neural tube defects was hypothesized as early as 1965; and in 1998, it became mandatory to add folic acid to cereal grains to address this public health threat.

Did you know? Although the fortification of food has greatly reduced the numbers of spina bifida cases, there is increasing evidence that deficiencies in folate and vitamin B_{12} still exist and are tied to increasing rates of dementia and congenital heart defects. Research has also indicted that low folate intake has resulted in poorer school performance for adolescents.

HOW MUCH IS ENOUGH?

The DV for folate is 400 mcg, based on a 2,000-calorie diet.

Dietary Reference Intakes (DRIs) for Vitamin B$_9$ (Folate)

Age	Children (mcg/day)	Males (mcg/day)	Females (mcg/day)	Pregnancy (mcg/day)	Lactation (mcg/day)
0–6 months	65				
6–12 months	80				
1–3 years	150				
4–8 years	200				
9–13 years		300	300		
14–18 years		400	400	600	500
19–50 years		400	400	600	500
51+ years		400	400		

SOURCE: Food and Nutrition Board, Institutes of Medicine, National Academies

Too much! Folate intake from food is generally not a concern, but when taking the better-absorbed folic acid, it can be a problem (see below). A tolerable UL has been set for 1,000 mcg of folic acid.

Supplement it? It is advised not to exceed 1,000 mcg of supplemental folic acid per day, as it may mask a B_{12} deficiency, which happens more in the elderly than in younger people. Most multivitamins contain adequate folic acid of 400 mcg and most contain adequate vitamin B_{12} as well.

First Place: Chicken Liver

For the full health benefits of chicken liver, see page 287. In a meta-analysis of fourteen studies, higher intake of folate-rich foods and higher blood levels of folate were associated with lower risk of coronary heart disease. Although chicken liver is the richest source of folate, this isn't the type of food the study was referring to, because the cardiovascular benefits of folate can be offset by the high cholesterol found in chicken liver. Advice? Limit to a 3-ounce serving once per week!

First Runner-Up: Lentils

For the full scoop of the health benefits of lentils, see page 289. Many studies have shown that the more folate in the diet the lower the risk of plugged-up arteries.

Second Runner-Up: Cowpeas

For more on the healthy properties of cowpeas, see page 287. A Penn State study revealed that only 7.9 percent of Americans are consuming legumes on any given day. Those who added ½ cup of legumes such as cowpeas per day made a significant contribution to not only their folate intake but also to their fiber, iron, magnesium, protein, and zinc stores, while lowering their intake of saturated fat and total fat.

Fourth: Pinto Beans

Besides being a great source of folate, pinto beans are an excellent source of fiber, iron, manganese, molybdenum, phosphorus, protein, and thiamine.

The most recent National Health and Nutrition Examination Survey found that, to no real surprise, we consume calorie-dense yet nutrient-poor foods in abundance. This is bad enough, but what was also discovered is that we choose to eat these foods in lieu of healthier foods. Translated: We eat more junk while sacrificing important nutrients, such as folate. The good news is that many companies are meeting people where they live by adding bean powders to familiar foods such as pasta to boost folate and other key nutrients naturally.

Fifth: Chickpeas

For more detail on the healthy properties of chickpeas, see page 287. Including folate-rich foods such as chickpeas may benefit mental illness and metabolic syndrome.

Sixth: Spinach

For the lowdown on this powerhouse veggie, see page 291. A study of pregnant Japanese women in their first trimester found that those who included spinach in their diet had the highest level of folate, which is important for fighting birth defects.

Shocker Food!

A cup of cooked asparagus supplies 253 mcg of folate, fairly close to spinach, the reigning king of folate in the green vegetable category. Asparagus is also an excellent source of iron, thiamine, and vitamin K, and a good source of fiber; niacin; phosphorus; riboflavin; vitamins A, B_6, C, and E; and zinc.

Seventh: Black Beans

For more info on black beans, see page 286. Researchers at the University of Florida found that inadequate folate intake was associated with an increased risk for hyperhomocysteinemia (high levels of the inflammatory marker homocysteine), which can lead to hardening of the arteries; damage to DNA that may increase the risk of cancer; and increased risk for cognitive decline, such as senile dementia and Alzheimer's disease. They recommended increasing folate intake in the elderly, beyond an appropriate multivitamin, by including naturally occurring folate-rich foods, such as black beans.

TOP 7 SOURCES OF CHOLINE

SNEAK-A-PEEK: RANKINGS AT A GLANCE

Ranking	Food	Serving	Amount (mg)
First Place	**Beef liver (cooked)**	**3 ounces**	**355**
First Runner-Up	**Braunschweiger**	**3 slices 3 ounces**	**215**
Second Runner-Up	**Eggs (cooked)**	**1 large**	**147**
Fourth	Veal (cooked)	3 ounces	120
Fifth	Sockeye salmon (cooked)	3 ounces	96
Sixth	Pork (cooked)	3 ounces	94
Seventh	Lamb (cooked)	3 ounces	92

SOURCE: USDA National Nutrient Database for Standard Reference, Release 24

Honorable mentions: Duck, turkey, tomato products

Best food groups: Meat, eggs, fish

What is choline and why is it so important? Choline is classified as a water-soluble essential nutrient that is part of the B-vitamin complex. It is found mainly in the lipids (fats) that make up cell membranes, and in chemical neurotransmitters that are responsible for signaling messages in the brain. Choline is also important for several of life's most basic functions, including liver metabolism and the transportation of other nutrients throughout the body. In pregnancy, it helps protect the fetus by keeping homocysteine, a toxic amino acid, in check. Choline is also essential in the creation of the neurotransmitter acetylcholine, which plays a role in memory and learning.

There aren't any known symptoms of choline deficiencies in humans; however, choline deficiencies have been associated with poor fat metabolism and utilization, fatty liver, nervous tissue damage, possible development of liver carcinomas, and poor cognition.

Did you know? Although choline has been around since man's first bite of food, its definition as a "nutrient" is fairly new. It was first discovered in

1862; however, choline wasn't recognized to be an essential part of every-day diet until 1998. It was at this time that the Institute of Medicine established a DRI for choline.

HOW MUCH IS ENOUGH?

Even though the body can produce some choline, it is not sufficient to meet the recommended needs; therefore, it must be consumed in the diet.

A DV for choline has not been established.

A Duke University study found that the perinatal period is the most critical time for adequate choline intake for optimal memory capacity and decreased risk for age-related memory decline.

Dietary Reference Intakes (DRIs) for Choline

Age	Children (mg/day)	Males (mg/day)	Females (mg/day)	Pregnancy (mg/day)	Lactation (mg/day)
0–6 months	125				
7–12 months	150				
1–3 years	200				
4–8 years	400				
9–13 years		375	375		
14–18 years		550	400	450	550
19–50 years		550	425	450	550
51+ years		550	425		

SOURCE: Food and Nutrition Board, Institutes of Medicine, National Academies

Too much! Consuming high amounts of choline can lead to an unusual, fishy body odor, increased sweating and salivation . . . even episodes of vomiting. These side effects have been observed at intakes of 10 to 15 g of choline, so make sure you stay below the tolerable UL of 3.5 g per day.

Supplement it? Choline can be found in supplements such as soy lecithin, a fatty substance that features both choline and the B vitamin inositol, which comes in capsules, liquid, or granular form; and as cytidine-5'-diphosphate (CPD) choline.

First Place: Beef Liver

For more info on the healthy properties of liver, see page 286. An interesting case-controlled study performed in Uruguay determined that consumption of white meat, poultry, fish, and liver might be protective against esophageal cancer. This certainly is not in side step with other studies that suggest increased red meat consumption may increase the risk of certain types of cancer. But this may be a good example of how all "red meats" may not be created equal. Of course, more research is needed.

First Runner-Up: Braunschweiger

For more info on this type of liverwurst, see page 290. A Johns Hopkins study found that postmenopausal women who had low choline intake in their diet were at much greater risk of developing fibrosis of the liver if they were diagnosed with nonalcoholic fatty liver disease. Without adequate choline, fat accumulates in the liver.

Second Runner-Up: Eggs

For more information on the "incredible edible" egg, see page 287. Eggs are an excellent source of choline. In addition, they are a good source of phosphorus, protein, riboflavin, and vitamin D.

An egg or two each day might be very beneficial for people with type 2 diabetes who are trying to improve their health. A study determined that incorporating two eggs per day in a high-protein, high-cholesterol diet has very positive results. Participants who were assigned to this diet experienced a 13-pound weight loss, along with improved glycemic control and a decrease in total cholesterol, while also experiencing an increase in HDL-cholesterol.

> In France, breaking an egg is considered good luck. Before stepping into their new home, French brides break an egg for good luck and healthy babies.

Shocker Food!

What do you add to cake mix to make cake? Eggs! Also the flour used to make cake is enriched with a number of nutrients. Bottom line: Although cake contains nutrients, including choline, it also brings along such undesirables as sugar, calories, and saturated fat, so don't think you can "have your cake and eat it, too" when it comes to turning to cake as a good source of nutrition. Treat cake for what it is—a treat! Have a small piece and move on!

Fourth: Veal

For more on the healthy properties of lean veal, see page 286. In a controlled study, Italian researchers found that compared with the control group, rats that were fed a choline-deficient diet were less capable of learning new tasks. Also discovered was that mitochondria in brain cells thrive on choline, which may play a role in cognition in rats as well as in humans.

Fifth: Sockeye Salmon

For more sock-it-to-you details on this fab fish, see page 291. A five-year study showed that consumption of fatty fish, including salmon, is associated with a reduced risk of impaired cognitive function. In addition to choline, omega-3 fatty acids have also been found to help with memory recall and proper brain function.

Sixth: Pork

For more on the benefits of lean pork, see page 290.

Seventh: Lamb

Leg of lamb is an excellent source of pantothenic acid, protein, selenium, vitamin B_{12}, and zinc, and a good source of iron and phosphorus.

TOP 7 SOURCES OF VITAMIN B_{12}

SNEAK-A-PEEK: RANKINGS AT A GLANCE

Ranking	Food	Serving	Amount (mcg)
First Place	Beef liver (cooked)	3 ounces	71
First Runner-Up	Clams (cooked)	3 ounces	16
Second Runner-Up	Braunschweiger	3 slices (3 ounces)	16
Fourth	Crab (cooked)	3 ounces	10
Fifth	Sardines (canned)	3 ounces	8
Sixth	Oysters (raw)	3 ounces	7
Seventh	Sockeye salmon (cooked)	3 ounces	5

SOURCE: USDA National Nutrient Database for Standard Reference, Release 24

Honorable mentions: Fortified cereals, chicken and turkey giblets

Best food groups: Meats, seafood, fortified foods

What is vitamin B_{12} and why is it so important? Vitamin B_{12} is a water-soluble vitamin. It exists in several forms that all contain the mineral cobalt; that is why they are collectively known as cobalamins. The main function of vitamin B_{12} is to act as a helper or cofactor for critical chemical reactions in the body that produce hormones, proteins, lipids, and red blood cells, and to ensure proper neurological function in the body. Deficiencies in vitamin B_{12}, caused by inadequate intake or due to health challenges, are often manifested as: megaloblastic anemia, loss of appetite, weight loss, fatigue/weakness, depression, dementia, and poor memory.

Did you know? The human body can store several years' worth of vitamin B_{12} in the liver. This is why deficiencies of this vitamin can be rarer compared to other nutritional deficiencies. However, a B_{12} deficiency is more likely to happen due to a lack of stomach acid and/or a substance present in the gut called intrinsic factor, which helps the vitamin absorb into the body. This is more common in the elderly.

HOW MUCH IS ENOUGH?

The DV for B_{12} is 6 mcg, based on a 2,000-calorie diet.

Dietary Reference Intakes (DRIs) for Vitamin B_{12}

Age	Children (mcg/day)	Males (mcg/day)	Females (mcg/day)	Pregnancy (mcg/day)	Lactation (mcg/day)
1–3 years	0.7				
4–8 years	1.0				
9–13 years		1.5	1.5		
14–18 years		2.0	2.0	2.2	2.4
19–50 years		2.0	2.0	2.2	2.4
51+ years		2.0	2.0		

Source: Food and Nutrition Board, IOM, National Academies

Too much! Vitamin B_{12} has a very low potential for toxicity. This, along with the fact that there are no adverse effects associated with excess vitamin B_{12} intake, has led the Institute of Medicine to not establish a UL for this nutrient. However, the DV for vitamin B_{12} is 6 mcg per day, which is nearly two and a half times higher than the RDA for adults.

Supplement it? Vitamin B_{12} is commonly added to fortified food, so by eating this food, you are in a way already being supplemented with this vitamin. However, vitamin B_{12} is commonly found in multivitamins, in vitamin B-complex supplements, or as a stand-alone supplements in tablet, capsule, and sublingual versions.

First Place: Beef Liver

For more info on the health benefits of beef liver, see page 286. Whether you go by DV or RDA, beef liver delivers an abundance of B_{12}. Keep in mind that the serving size is 3 ounces. You could easily reduce the portion size to 2 ounces, which would provide about 48 mcg of vitamin B_{12} and 216 mg of cholesterol.

First Runner-Up. Clams

Clams are an excellent source of iron, manganese, selenium, and vitamin B_{12}, and a good source of copper, phosphorus, riboflavin, and vitamin C.

Don't really like the consistency of clams? Not to worry: A study suggested that the broth of canned clams contains high amounts of vitamin B_{12}. Up to 72 percent of the clams' vitamin B_{12} can be recovered from the broth! An animal study demonstrated cholesterol reduction in rats that were fed clam extract.

Second Runner-Up: Braunschweiger

For more info on the health properties of this sausage, see page 290. What's so unique about braunschweiger is that those who don't care for liver may actually like this spreadable form.

Fourth: Crab

Depending on the type of crab, edible meat that you are able to extract from crab ranges anywhere from 10 to 25 percent of the whole crab weight. Crabs are an excellent source of copper, selenium, vitamin B_{12}, and zinc; and a good source of iron, magnesium, niacin, and phosphorus, riboflavin, and vitamin C.

New research is showing there is an inverse relationship between eating shellfish, crab included, and the risk of developing type 2 diabetes. This means the higher consumption of shellfish, the lower the risk is of developing type 2 diabetes.

Fifth: Sardines

Sardines, the first fish to ever be canned, are an excellent source of calcium, niacin, omega-3, phosphorus, selenium, and vitamins B_{12} and D. They are also a good source of iron, vitamins B_2 and B_6, and zinc.

Fish consumption has many benefits; however, there might also be some risks, too. A recent study indicated that the benefits—reduction of coronary heart disease, decrease of mild hypertension, prevention of certain cardiac arrhythmias, and sudden death—outweighed the risk of ingesting contaminants found in the fish. Sardines, because they are very small, have the least amount of contaminants and are safer to eat compared to other fish.

Sixth: Oysters

Cooked oysters are an excellent source of copper, iron, and selenium, vitamin B_{12}, and zinc. They are also a good source of magnesium, phosphorus, and riboflavin.

A team of researchers from the United States and Italy found that oysters contain two compounds that have shown in animal studies to stimulate the release of testosterone and estrogen. This may affirm that oysters may help libido after all!

Although some food oysters can produce pearls, they should not be confused with pearl oysters, which belong to a different bivalve family. Oysters change gender several times over the course of their lifetime. They are also natural water filtration systems: one adult oyster can filter more than 60 gallons of water a day!

Seventh: Sockeye Salmon

For more info on this piscatory powerhouse, see page 291. Low maternal B_{12} levels during pregnancy have been linked to increased infant crying. And a baby who cries all the time could get pretty depressing. Interestingly, low levels of omega-3 fatty acids have also been tied to postpartum depression, so eating two servings of sockeye salmon each week may be just the two-fer for a happy mom and baby!

Shocker Food! ——————————————

There aren't many vegetarian sources of vitamin B_{12}, but nutritional yeast, which is grown on blackstrap molasses, contains an active form of the vitamin. It comes as yellow flakes or powder and has a nice cheese flavor; it is wonderful sprinkled on top of popcorn. About 2 rounded teaspoons of nutritional yeast provides the recommended amount of vitamin B_{12} for adults.

TOP 7 SOURCES OF VITAMIN C

SNEAK-A-PEEK: RANKINGS AT A GLANCE

Ranking	Food	Serving	Amount (mg)
First Place	Guava	1 cup	376
First Runner-Up	Sweet red peppers (cooked) Red peppers (raw)	1 cup 1 cup	233 190
Second Runner-Up	Kiwi	1 cup	167
Fourth	Orange juice	1 cup	124
Fifth	Hot green peppers (raw) Green peppers (cooked)	1 cup 1 cup	120 101
Sixth	Broccoli (cooked)	1 cup	101
Seventh	Strawberries	1 cup	98

SOURCE: USDA National Nutrient Database for Standard Reference, Release 24

Honorable mentions: Grapefruit juice, kohlrabi, papayas, Brussels sprouts

Best food groups: Vegetables, fruits

What is vitamin C why is it so important? Human beings need to consume a vitamin C source each and every day because it's neither made nor stored in the body. It is a powerful antioxidant that helps protect against free radical damage that can lead to aging, heart disease, cancer, and the list goes on and on. Vitamin C is also vital to the formation of collagen, a protein found in skin, tendons, cartilage, bones, and teeth. Signs of vitamin C deficiency include bleeding gums and loose teeth, nosebleeds and easy bruising, poor wound healing, and increased susceptibility to infections. A vitamin C deficiency disease called scurvy was commonly seen in sailors who embarked on long ocean voyages until in the mid-eighteenth century it was discovered that citrus fruits could prevent the disease. Today it is rarely seen except in elderly people who are malnourished. The word *ascorbic*, as in ascorbic acid (the chemical name for vitamin C), means "no scurvy."

Did you know? All mammals, with the exception of some monkeys, guinea pigs, Indian fruit-eating bats, and humans, can make their own vitamin C.

HOW MUCH IS ENOUGH?

The DV for vitamin C is 90 mg, based on a 2,000-calorie diet.

Dietary Reference Intakes (DRIs) for Vitamin C

Age	Children (mg/day)	Males (mg/day)	Females (mg/day)	Pregnancy (mg/day)	Lactation (mg/day)
0–6 months	40				
7–12 months	50				
1–3 years	15				
4–8 years	25				
9–13 years		45	45		
14–18 years		75	65	80	115
19–70 years		90	75	85	120

SOURCE: Food and Nutrition Board, Institutes of Medicine, National Academies

Too much! The UL is set at 2,000 mg, but even higher levels are known to be well tolerated in healthy individuals. Diarrhea is often the first indication that an excess level has been reached in the body and that its time to back off. Large doses of vitamin C have been associated with higher risk of developing kidney stones, too.

One of the unique benefits of vitamin C is that it can help increase iron absorption from food. That's a bad thing if you have blood disorders that produce too much iron in your system, such as hemochromatosis.

Supplement it? Adequate vitamin C levels can be achieved easily through diet. However, if additional vitamin C is needed or you find it difficult to meet your needs through food sources, a supplement may be appropriate for you. Ascorbic acid comes in powder, tablets, capsules, chewables, and liquids. Buffered and time-released forms are also available.

First Place: Guavas

One cup of guava supplies four times what you need in a day of vitamin C! Guava comes in many shapes, sizes, and flavors. The flesh of the fruit is sweet and fragrant and ranges in color from white, yellow, and pink to red. The strawberry guava is quite popular but not as high in vitamin C as other varieties. Guava is also an excellent source of fiber, folate, lycopene, and vitamin A, and a good source of potassium and vitamin A. Guava also contains a vast amount of plant nutrients, such as essential oils, flavonoids, lectins, phenols, saponins, triterpenes, and tannins.

Studies showed that guava sends messages to cancer cells that their days are numbered by increasing apoptosis (programmed cell death) and preventing the spread of malignant cells.

First Runner-Up: Sweet Red Peppers

Besides providing vitamin C, red peppers are also an excellent source of vitamin A and a good source of folate, lycopene, and other carotenoids. Hot pepper varieties are cherished for their thermogenic (fat-burning) effect in the body. But a Japanese study showed that the sweet red bell pepper had similar thermogenic properties without creating all that heat in the mouth. Sweet red varieties were also shown to block pain receptors in a similar fashion to that of hot red peppers!

Second Runner-Up: Kiwis

Kiwis are considered one of the most nutrient-dense fruits on the planet. Besides being an excellent source of vitamin C, they are also rich in fiber and a good source of folate and potassium. In a Chinese study, subjects

> Kiwi was originally known as the Chinese gooseberry, until Norman Sondag, an American importer, remarked how closely the fruit resembled the New Zealand kiwi bird.

who suffered from the constipation type of irritable bowel syndrome (IBS) ate two kiwis in addition to their regular diet for four weeks. The majority of the group experienced more frequent bowel movements and shorter bowel transit time (less time between eating and having a bowel movement).

Fourth: Orange Juice

To pulp or not to pulp . . . that is the question. Research confirms that orange juice with pulp is healthier than the reduced-pulp or pulp-free versions. In addition to being a terrific source of vitamin C, OJ is also a good source of folate and potassium. Orange juice is rich in the plant nutrient hesperidin, which is mainly found in the pulp and white fleshy underbelly of the skin of the orange. Hesperidin was found to be helpful in lowering blood pressure and improving the health of arteries. Regular consumption of OJ also reduced inflammation and reduced risk factors for developing hardening of the arteries.

Fifth: Hot Peppers

Hot peppers, if measured by the cup like the other vegetables in this book, would have ranked first runner-up! But, seriously, can you eat a cup? They are also a good source of vitamin A. Green chile peppers contain the plant nutrient capsaicin, which has strong antibacterial activity. This may explain why spicy foods have a long tradition in hot climates, where modern refrigeration was not always available to prevent food from spoiling. Capsaicin is also useful in controlling pain. A double-blind study looked at capsaicin's being applied to the surgical site in patients who received total knee replacements. Significantly less opioid medications were needed postsurgery, better ambulation was experienced, and much lower pain scores were reported in the capsaicin treatment group, compared to the placebo group that received standard postoperative care.

Sixth: Broccoli

Broccoli belongs to the cruciferous family of vegetables that include cabbage, cauliflower, kale collard greens, and Brussels sprouts. Broccoli is an excellent source of vitamin K and also a good source of folate and vitamins A and B$_6$.

Broccoli reigns supreme in its cancer-fighting plant chemicals (glucosinolate) content, compared to other cruciferous cousins. However, regular consumption of any kind of cruciferous vegetables may reduce the risk of prostate, breast, lung, and colorectal cancers.

Seventh: Strawberries

Besides being rich in vitamin C, strawberries are also a good source of folate and many plant nutrients, such as anthocyanins, catechins, ellagic acid, and flavonoids. Fisetin, a flavonoid found abundantly in strawberries, may help fight a variety of cancer types, including breast, prostate, cervical, and melanoma, as well as also fighting depression and improving cognitive function. A randomized double-blind study using freeze-dried strawberry powder found that those subjects who consumed the equivalent of four servings of frozen strawberries had the greatest reduction in risk factors associated with obesity, such as stroke, diabetes, and cardiovascular disease.

TOP 7 SOURCES OF VITAMIN D

SNEAK-A-PEEK: RANKINGS AT A GLANCE

Ranking	Food	Serving	Amount (IU)
First Place	Rainbow trout (cooked)	3 ounces	16.2
First Runner-Up	Sockeye, pink, or Chinook salmon (cooked)	3 ounces	11.1–14.5
Second Runner-Up	Swordfish (cooked)	3 ounces	14.1
Fourth	Tuna, light (canned)	3 ounces	5.7
Fifth	Halibut (cooked)	3 ounces	4.9
Sixth	Sardines (cooked)	3 ounces	4.1
Seventh	Rockfish (cooked)	3 ounces	3.9

SOURCE: USDA National Nutrient Database for Standard Reference, Release 24

Honorable mentions: Fortified milk and other fortified foods, beef liver, shrimp, egg yolks, mushrooms

Best food groups: Fatty fish, meat, eggs, dairy

Ultimate best source: The sun!

What is vitamin D and why is it so important? Vitamin D is really not a vitamin; rather, it is a hormone made by the body in response to the exposure of skin to sunlight. Whether it comes from sunlight or the food you eat, it must be converted into an active form that the body can use, called calcitriol. We need vitamin D for the maintenance of strong bones and teeth and the prevention of rickets, a disease characterized by soft, thin, and brittle bones. The vitamin helps the body absorb calcium from food and it is required to coax the immune system into action. Without adequate amounts of vitamin D in the body, a part of the immune system called T cells remains dormant and unresponsive to invading viruses and bacteria. Inadequate vitamin D intake may also be linked to a such conditions as heart disease, diabetes, multiple sclerosis (MS), high blood pressure, certain types of cancer, and depression.

HOW MUCH IS ENOUGH?

The DV for vitamin D is 400 IU, based on a 2,000-calorie diet.

Dietary Reference Intakes (DRIs) for Vitamin D

Age	Children (IU/day)	Males (IU/day)	Females (IU/day)	Pregnancy (IU/day)	Lactation (IU/day)
0–12 months	400				
1–13 years	600				
14–18 years		600	600		
19–70 years		600	600	600	600
71+ years		800	800		

SOURCE: Food and Nutrition Board, Institutes of Medicine, National Academies

Many experts contend the recently revised DRI is still far too low and only addresses bone health and not other medical conditions. In multiple sclerosis, higher levels of vitamin D were associated with lower risk of developing the disease. High levels are also associated with lower relapse rates.

Too much! The UL established for vitamin D is 4,000 IU; however, levels far above that have been known to be well tolerated for short periods of time. Signs of vitamin D toxicity include loss of appetite; weight loss; frequent urination; abnormal heart rhythm; and hypocalcaemia (high calcium), which can harden the circulatory system and organs in the body.

Everyone agrees that overexposure to the sun is not a good thing, but oddly enough, it is *not* one of the causes of vitamin D toxicity. The heat given off the skin limits the amount of vitamin D your body will absorb.

Supplement it? You'll find vitamin D supplements in a variety of multivitamins and bone-building formulations. Individual vitamin D supplements come in two different forms, D_2 (ergocalciferol, a vegetarian source) and D_3 (cholecalciferol, from animal sources), and can be found in liquid, capsule, tablet, and chewable forms. About ten minutes in the midday summer sun, clad in a bathing suit but minus the sunscreen, is thought to produce about 10,000 IU of vitamin D for fair-skinned people. The elderly and darker-skinned individuals don't produce as much vitamin D from UV ray exposure.

First Place: Rainbow Trout

For a rainbow of information on the healthy properties of trout, see page 292. A review of thirteen studies revealed that eating a serving of fatty fish, such as trout, only once a week could reduce your risk of dying from heart disease by 15 percent. If you added in another 5-ounce serving, total risk was reduced the risk by 22 percent!

You no longer have to don your waders, grab your fly-fishing gear, and head out west to enjoy a delicious dinner of rainbow trout. There are over eight hundred trout-rearing farms in the United States.

First Runner-Up: Sockeye Salmon, Pink, and Chinook

In addition to being a great source of vitamin D, Chinook salmon is an excellent source of niacin and protein, and a good source of omega-3 fatty acids and selenium. Pink and sockeye salmon (see page 291) are runners-up to this runner-up, in terms of vitamin E content. A study that looked at the blood of women who ate two servings of salmon/week found that they had superior antioxidant protection status compared to those women who ate fewer. Higher vitamin A and selenium levels were observed in the two-servings/week group.

> Chinook (or king) salmon is not only the largest of the salmon family, with mature adults commonly exceeding 40 pounds and some reportedly as large as 120 pounds, but is also the state fish of Alaska.

Second Runner-Up: Swordfish

For more info on this fish with the sword-shaped snout, sure see page 291. No doubt about it . . . swordfish is quite nutritious. However, because of its large size and predatory nature, methyl mercury accumulation is a concern with swordfish consumption and the FDA and the EPA have advised pregnant women and children not to eat it.

Fourth: Tuna, Light

The term *light tuna* actually refers to a combination of species of tuna that are lighter in appearance such as skipjack, yellowfin, tongol, and bigeye. Light tuna varieties are lower in mercury than albacore and are an excellent source of niacin, phosphorus, and vitamins B_6, B_{12}, and D; and a good source of iron. The cornerstone of a healthy Mediterranean diet is fatty fish, such as tuna. A review of several studies showed that the risk of having a stroke was fairly significant for those who ate fatty fish once a week. However, those who ate fatty fish five or more times each week had a 31 percent reduced risk of stroke. Elderly subjects who consumed tuna fish had less strokes and more normal MRI scans of the brain.

Fifth: Halibut

Halibut are an excellent source of magnesium, niacin, phosphorus, protein, selenium, and vitamin D, and a good source of omega 3-fats and vitamin B_{12}. In a study of rats that were fed selenium from a variety of dietary sources, halibut proved most efficient in restoring depleted stores out of any food tested.

Sixth: Sardines

For more on this small fish (one of the safest sources of fish for pregnant women), see page 291.

Vitamin D plays a very important role in pregnancy, especially in the development of fetal bone health. However, in a study that looked at consumption trends in pregnant women, fewer than 25 percent of those women consumed vitamin D–rich fatty fish, such as sardines.

Seventh: Rockfish

Besides providing vitamin D, a 3-ounce portion of rockfish is also an excellent source of choline and selenium, and a good source of potassium. A study conducted in the United Kingdom found that vitamin D status was best in meat and fish eaters, compared to vegan and vegetarians.

Shocker Food!

Nutritionally, white button and brown portobello mushrooms compare well to the more expensive shiitake mushroom, though shiitakes are higher in vitamin E and polyunsaturated fatty acids. Much like human skin, mushrooms exposed to ultraviolet light can generate large amounts of vitamin D_2. Dole, of pineapple and banana fame, has ramped up this process by drying and grinding portobello mushrooms before exposing them to UV rays. This greatly increases their surface area and their vitamin D production. One teaspoon of the dried mushroom powder provides 600 IU of vitamin D, enough to meet the needs of a vegan.

TOP 7 SOURCES OF VITAMIN E

SNEAK-A-PEEK: RANKINGS AT A GLANCE

Ranking	Food	Serving	Amount (IU)
First Place	Almonds	1 ounce	7.43
First Runner-Up	Sunflower seeds (roasted)	1 ounce	7.4
Second Runner-Up	Spinach (cooked)	1 cup	6.7
Fourth	Sunflower oil	1 tablespoon	5.6
Fifth	Safflower oil	1 tablespoon	4.6
Sixth	Turnip greens (cooked)	1 cup	4.4
Seventh	Hazelnuts	1 ounce	4.3

SOURCE: USDA National Nutrient Database for Standard Reference, Release 24

Honorable mentions: Fortified cereals, potato chips, mixed nuts, tomato paste and pasta sauce

Best food groups: Nuts, seeds, vegetables

What is vitamin E and why is it so important? Vitamin E is like a moat to a castle: Its job is to put up a protective barrier to safeguard against foreign invaders. In the body's case, that invader is a rogue group called free radicals. No . . . not a hippie group from the '60s; rather, toxic substances in the body that are hell-bent on maiming and destroying every cell of your body. Free radical damage paves the way to aging, heart disease, cancer, diabetes, and the list goes on. Vitamin E puts a serious hurt on free radicals by functioning as an antioxidant. It is also essential for maintaining immune system, heart, and eye health. Research has shown that vitamin E might lower the incidence of cataracts and help prevent heart disease, to boot!

Did you know? There are actually eight chemical forms of vitamin E, which fall into two different groups. The groups are called tocotrienols and tocopherols. Within these groups are four different forms of the vitamin. The only form of vitamin E that is biologically active in the human body is alpha-tocopherol.

HOW MUCH IS ENOUGH?

The DV for vitamin E is 30 IU, based on a 2,000-calorie diet.

Dietary Reference Intakes (DRIs) for Vitamin E

Age	Children (IU/day)	Males (IU/day)	Females (IU/day)	Pregnancy (IU/day)	Lactation (IU/day)
0–6 months	6				
7–12 months	7.5				
1–3 years	9				
4–8 years	10.4				
9–13 years		16.4	16.4		
14–18 years		22.4	22.4	22.4	28.4
19+ years		22.4	22.4	22.4	28.4

SOURCE: Food and Nutrition Board, Institutes of Medicine, National Academies

Too much! The tolerable UL of vitamin E has been set at 1,500 IU per day. Toxicity symptoms have been observed with vitamin E supplementation of 3,000 IU per day for three months. The most common symptom of vitamin E toxicity is hemorrhage, but toxicity can also manifest as nausea, diarrhea, muscle weakness, and overall fatigue.

Supplement it? Vitamin E supplements come in form of alpha-tocopherol, which makes sense since this form is the most biologically active. A large randomized placebo controlled study revealed that there may be increased risk of prostate cancer when vitamin E supplementation of 400 IU per day was used. Other research has shown mixed results for supplementing with vitamin E.

First Place: Almonds

Almonds are an excellent source of magnesium, manganese (30 percent of the DV per serving), protein, and vitamin E (35 percent of the DV per serving), plus a good source of copper, fiber, phosphorus, and vitamin B_2. Ounce for ounce, almonds are the tree nut highest in calcium, fiber, niacin, protein, riboflavin, and vitamin E. Worried about controlling your blood glucose level? A small study showed adding one to two handfuls of almonds to a high-carbohydrate meal helped control blood glucose better. Almond consumption is also associated with reducing LDL cholesterol and aiding weight management.

> There are over thirty types of almonds; the Nonpareil is the most popular in the United States.

First Runner-Up: Sunflower Seeds

Sunflower seeds are very nutritious and an excellent source of copper, magnesium, selenium, and vitamins B_1 and E. They are also a good source of folate, phosphorus, and vitamin B_6. Sunflower seeds rank number three in plant phytosterols (see page 133 for a complete listing), a compound that can help reduce cholesterol levels.

Second Runner-Up: Spinach

For more on the healthy properties of Popeye's favorite, see page 291. Besides containing a hefty amount of vitamin E, spinach is also known to produce nitric oxide, which helps improve blood pressure. A randomized, controlled crossover trial of a group of healthy men and women looked at the effects of eating spinach on a variety and health indicators. Compared to the control group, those who ate spinach experienced several health benefits, including lower blood pressure.

Fourth: Sunflower Oil

Besides being rich in vitamin E, the mid-oleic (standard) and high-oleic varieties of this oil are rich in monounsaturated fats, which help keep cholesterol in check. The study comparing olive oil and mid-oleic sunflower oil showed that individuals experienced significantly lower total cholesterol and LDL cholesterol than those on the sunflower oil diet.

> High-oleic (also called high-stearic) sunflower oil has a higher smoke point, lending this oil to more applications for replacing solid fats in baking, frying, and so on.

Fifth: Safflower oil

Safflowers were originally grown because the flowers were used to make red and yellow dyes for clothing and food preparation. Now, safflowers are primarily grown for oil production. With its composition of 8 percent saturated fat, 15 percent polyunsaturated fat, and 77 percent monounsaturated fats and its being a good source of vitamin E, safflower oil makes a terrific cooking oil. In addition, safflower oil has shown promise in the battle of the bulge. In a study of obese postmenopausal women with type 2 diabetes, those who supplemented their diet with safflower oil for 32 weeks had reduced fat around the midsection, increased muscle growth, lowered fasting blood sugar, and increase in a hormone called adiponectin, whose job is to improve insulin sensitivity.

Shocker Food!

A standard portion of 1 ounce of potato chips contains 3.23 IU of vitamin E, or more than 10 percent of its DV! No, potatoes aren't really that great of a source of vitamin E—but the oils that the chips are cooked in are. So crunch n moderation!

Sixth: Turnip Greens

Don't discard your turnip tops—they are an excellent source of folate, manganese, and vitamins A and C. In addition, they are a good source of copper, fiber, and vitamins B_6 and E. The Brassica (cruciferous) vegetable family, as a rule, contains many nutrients that help safeguard your health, such as glucosinolates and phenolics. Turnip greens rank among the top for these compounds.

Seventh: Hazelnuts

Hazelnuts (also known as filberts) are an excellent source of copper and manganese. In addition, they are a good source of vitamin E, fiber, and magnesium. Hazelnuts can help reduce cholesterol. A recent study showed that fifteen men with high cholesterol who ate about thirty hazelnuts (40 g) per day experienced a decrease in components of LDL cholesterol and an increase in HDL.

TOP 7 SOURCES OF VITAMIN K

SNEAK-A-PEEK: RANKINGS AT A GLANCE

Ranking	Food	Serving	Amount (mcg)
First Place	Kale (cooked)	1 cup	1,147
First Runner-Up	Collard greens (cooked)	1 cup	1,059
Second Runner-Up	Spinach (cooked)	1 cup	1,027
Fourth	Turnip greens (cooked)	1 cup	851
Fifth	Beet greens (cooked)	1 cup	697
Sixth	Dandelion greens (cooked)	1 cup	579
Seventh	Swiss chard (cooked)	1 cup	572

SOURCE: USDA National Nutrient Database for Standard Reference, Release 24

Honorable mentions: Brussels sprouts, parsley, broccoli, asparagus

Best food groups: Green leafy vegetables

What is vitamin K and why is it so important? Without it, our body would be one big bruise! Vitamin K is integral to what is called the blood-clotting cascade (coagulation) which prevents constant bleeding when we cut ourselves and internal hemorrhaging. Vitamin K is also extremely important in bone formation and in the prevention of osteoporosis. People who are on blood-thinning medications, such as Coumadin (warfarin), are often advised to limit their intake of foods rich in vitamin K. But research shows that having regular intake of vitamin K helps the body exert better control of the anticoagulation effect of the medicine and balance it with clotting needed in the body. The key is having a consistent intake of vitamin K–rich foods, which helps the doctor better regulate the anticoagulant medication.

Did you know? Vitamin K actually refers to a group of fat-soluble vitamins: K_1, also known as phylloquinone, comes from plant sources; and K_2, which refers to a subgroup called menaquinones, comes from animal sources and the synthesis of intestinal bacteria.

> The *K* in *vitamin K* came from a German medical journal, where it was referred to as *Koagulationsvitamin*.

HOW MUCH IS ENOUGH?

The DV for vitamin K is 80 mcg, based on a 2,000-calorie diet.

Dietary Reference Intakes (DRIs) for Vitamin K

Age	Children (mcg/day)	Males (mcg/day)	Females (mcg/day)	Pregnancy (mcg/day)	Lactation (mcg/day)
0–6 months	2				
6–12 months	2.5				
1–3 years	30				
4–8 years	55				
9–13 years		60	60		
14–18 years		75	75	75	75
19–50 years		120	90	90	90
51+ years		120	90		

SOURCE: Food and Nutrition Board, Institutes of Medicine, National Academies

Too much! An UL for vitamin K hasn't been established. Consuming high amounts of vitamin K via food sources generally doesn't pose a problem. However, high intake of vitamin K supplements has been known to cause liver damage and jaundice. Again, if you are prescribed blood thinners, be sure to discuss your dietary intake of this vitamin with your doctor.

Supplement it? Vitamin K can be found in multivitamins or as a supplement alone. Supplementing vitamin K has been showed to increase bone density and reduce bone loss and fractures.

First Place: Kale

For the skinny on kale, see page 288. Kale belongs to the cruciferous vegetable family, a category of vegetables linked to cancer prevention. High intake of cruciferous vegetables, such as kale, has been related to reduced risk of both breast and prostate cancer.

First Runner-Up: Collard Greens

For the amazing nutritional profile of collards, see page 288. For best cholesterol-lowering benefits, make sure to cook your collards. A study found that cooked versus raw collards did a much better job on binding cholesterol contained in the digestive system.

Second Runner-Up: Spinach

There are different varieties of spinach, ranging from flat leaves, smooth leaves, to savory, crinkled leaves. Baby spinach is usually flat-leafed. For more info on the many benefits of Olive Oyl's boyfriend's favorite treat, see page 291. Spinach was shown to help improve blood flow and lower blood pressure in a randomized control study. The flavonoids and nitrates in spinach help produce nitric acid, which helps open up blood vessels.

Fourth: Turnip Greens

Turnip greens are the green leafy portion of the turnip, a root vegetable in the mustard family that was originally brought to the United States by colonists. For detail on the nutrient profile of these greens, see page 288. Turnip greens contain glucoraphanin, a plant chemical that produces sulforaphane, a potent anticancer substance.

Shocker Food!

Onions may not be what first comes to mind when you think of a "leafy green," but they do provide over twice the RDA for vitamin K per cup serving. They also contain the flavonoid quercetin and other phyto-chemicals, which have been shown to protect against cancer, lower high blood pressure, and reduce the risk of heart attack.

Fifth: Beet Greens

Beet greens are very similar to turnip greens in that they are the sprout that comes up from the top of the root. They are an excellent source of vitamins A, C, and K, and a good source of riboflavin. An animal study found that mice that were fed a high-fat, high-cholesterol diet could prevent lipid peroxidation and improve antioxidant status when their diet was supplemented with beet greens.

Sixth: Dandelion Greens

Dandelion greens are an excellent source of vitamins A, C, and K, and a good source of calcium. Dandelion flowers are commonly used to make wine. Dandelions have traditionally been used in different medical systems from around the world, includ-

> The word *dandelion* originates from the French phrase *dent de lion*, "lion's tooth," inspired by the jagged appearance of the plant's leaves.

ing Native American and Arabic medicine. Extracts of dandelion have been shown to have antiviral and anti-influenza properties.

Seventh: Swiss Chard

Swiss chard is a member of the beet family, with the difference that the bulb it produces is not edible. Swiss chard is packed with 961 mg, or 27 percent, of the DV of potassium, which helps regulate blood pressure. It is also rich in iron, magnesium, and vitamins A, C, and K, and a good source of calcium and fiber. However, you might wish to watch your intake if watching your sodium; Swiss chard boasts one of the highest-occurring levels of sodium of all vegetables, with 313 mg per cup cooked.

Scientists in Urbino, Italy, discovered a flavonoid substance called xylosylvitexin in Swiss chard leaves and seeds, which inhibits the growth and duplication of human colon cancer cells. Another interesting fact is that it's not really "Swiss" at all, but originated in Sicily—a Swiss botanist named it after his beloved Switzerland.

CHAPTER 2

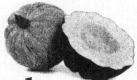

Digging the Minerals

TOP 7 SOURCES OF CALCIUM

SNEAK-A-PEEK: RANKINGS AT A GLANCE

Ranking	Food	Serving	Amount (mcg)
First Place	Hard cheese (Parmesan is highest)	1.5 ounces	300–468
First Runner-Up	Yogurt	1 cup	452
Second Runner-Up	Collard greens (cooked)	1 cup	357
Fourth	Rhubarb* (cooked)	1 cup	348
Fifth	Sardines (canned)	3 ounces	325
Sixth	Milk	1 cup	299–305
Seventh	Spinach* (cooked)	½ cup	291

*The bioavailability (your body's ability to absorb a nutrient) of calcium from plant foods is less than that from animal foods. That may be a more important factor than which foods contain more. Consuming a vitamin C source with these plant foods can help increase their calcium's bioavailability.
SOURCE: USDA National Nutrient Database for Standard Reference, Release 24

Honorable mentions: Soybeans, tofu, dark green vegetable sprouts, cauliflower, sesame seeds, red beans, Brazil nuts, herring, herbs

Best food groups: Dairy, green vegetables, soybeans, nuts and seeds, fish

What is calcium and why is it so important? Calcium is the fifth-most-abundant element found in nature. It is what makes up limestone and marble, coral, seashells and eggshells, antlers and bones. Our very structure depends on it, as 99 percent of all calcium stored in the body can be found in the bones (including teeth). It is also responsible for cardiovascular, nervous, and muscular cell conduction.

Lifestyle choices are the biggest contributor to calcium deficiencies: poor intake, lack of exercise, and tobacco or excessive alcohol use. Being underweight might cause more loss of calcium than being overweight; and hormonal imbalances, such as menopause, have also been found to disrupt calcium balance. Besides inadequate intake, calcium deficiencies can also be caused by certain diseases such as Crohn's, liver, and celiac disease. Health conditions associated with immobility or bed rest for more than six months, such as stroke, Parkinson's disease, or multiple sclerosis (MS), can waste calcium. Even certain medications, such as steroids, can deplete calcium.

When calcium is not adequate in your bloodstream, your body pulls it from its storage depots—a.k.a. your bones and teeth—which can lead to osteoporosis and dental problems. In addition, disorders of calcium deficiency can include congestive heart disorder, heart arrhythmias, hypotension, and muscle stiffness and cramps.

Did you know? Adequate calcium intake has been found to lower the risk of developing obesity, hypertension, hyperinsulinemia, and insulin resistance. Adequate vitamin D levels also help ensure appropriate calcium absorption (see page 45 for the best sources of vitamin D). Watch that sodium! It can compete with calcium for absorption in the body, meaning that too much sodium could contribute to the development of osteoporosis!

HOW MUCH IS ENOUGH?

The DV for calcium is 1,000 mg, based on a 2,000-calorie diet.

Dietary Reference Intakes (DRIs) for Calcium

Age	Males (mg/day)	Females (mg/day)	Pregnancy (mg/day)	Lactation (mg/day)
0–6 months	200	200		
7–12 months	260	260		
1–3 years	700	700		

continues

continued

Age	Males (mg/day)	Females (mg/day)	Pregnancy (mg/day)	Lactation (mg/day)
4–8 years	1,000	1,000		
9–13 years	1,300	1,300		
14–18 years	1,300	1,300	1,300	1,300
19–50 years	1,000	1,000	1,000	1,000
51–70 years	1,000	1,200		
71+ years	1,200	1,200		

SOURCE: Food and Nutrition Board, Institutes of Medicine, National Academies

Too much! Consuming excess calcium can lead to a buildup of calcium (hypercalcemia). Symptoms of hypercalcemia include fatigue, weakness, loss of appetite, nausea, excessive urination, dehydration, lethargy, stupor, and coma. Long-term calcium overload can lead to such health conditions as hyperparathyroidism, certain cancers, hyperthyroidism, hypervitaminosis D, immobilization, and sarcoidosis.

Supplement it? Considering that dairy products supply 78 percent of the calcium in the U.S. diet, it may be hard to maintain adequate calcium levels without consuming dairy or fortified foods. (Blood tests are *not* the best way to determine whether you have adequate stores of calcium in your body. Your body will leach calcium from your bones to keep blood levels normal if there are not adequate amounts of calcium in your diet. Ask your doctor if a bone density study may be in order.) Calcium can be found in multivitamins, bone formulations, by itself or in combinations with other nutrients.

First Place: Hard Cheese

Hard cheeses in general contain the most calcium of all the cheeses. Parmesan is made from partially skimmed cow's milk and typically aged anywhere from ten months to several years. The long aging process is what produces the crumbliness of Parmesan cheese. It is an excellent source of calcium and protein and a good source of phosphorous. In fact, cheeses are among the

Parmesan cheese dates back in the literature as early as the fourteenth century. Its namesake is Parma, one of five provinces in Italy that boast over 1,600 cheese factories.

most concentrated protein sources found on Earth, with Parmesan cheese containing more than 38 g of protein per 3.5 ounces of grated cheese. That is more than all meats and other protein sources.

First Runner-Up: Yogurt

For the full scoop on yogurt, turn to page 292. Three servings of yogurt per day given to women who had very poor calcium intake significantly slowed down the excretion of a chemical in the body that signals bone loss.

Second Runner-Up: Collard Greens

Got Collards? True—you don't see green mustache campaigns promoting collard greens for their calcium. However, get this: Cup for cup, collards have more calcium than milk! But when it comes to nutrient supremacy, it's what get's absorbed that matters. Unfortunately, green leafies, such as collards, are also high in oxalates, which can block some of the calcium from being absorbed. Serving dark greens with a vitamin C source such as a citrus glaze, or adorned with slices of citrus, can help. For more about the many benefits of collards, go to page 288.

Calcium-starved rats were attracted to the taste of collards over three other not-as-calcium-rich sources presented to them in a study. Calcium may contribute to the bitterness in greens and can be a turn-off to some humans. But if prepared the right way, the bitter flavor can be masked and acceptable to humans and rats alike!

Fourth: Rhubarb

The most popular use of rhubarb is in rhubarb pie or to make tarts and sauces. It is not naturally sweet, so sugar must be added. It is also a great source of fiber and a fair source of many other nutrients. Rhubarb is rich in calcium but also in oxalates, which can impede much of its calcium from being absorbed. It must also be prepared carefully (the rest of the plant, aside from the stalks, is poisonous). Bottom line? Enjoy it but don't count on it as a preferable source of calcium.

> The use of rhubarb as a medicinal plant dates back as far as 2700 BC in China, and supposedly it was given to the Wu emperor of the Liang dynasty to break a fever. In America, it is thought that a gardener from the state of Maine first planted rhubarb in the late 1700s after obtaining the seeds from Europe.

Fifth: Sardines

Sardines contain a boatload of soft bones (but you'd be hard pressed to feel them when you eat them because they are soft), which makes this food one of the best sources of calcium, provided you eat them with their bones. Sharing that vessel are many other nutrients; see page 291 to learn more about them. Along with dairy products, sardines are the main dietary source of calcium among the elderly. Unfortunately, they don't consume enough of these inexpensive little fishies to meet their needs and offset osteopenia and osteoporosis.

Sixth: Milk

No other naturally occurring drink contains as many nutrients as milk, which is the largest contributor of calcium, potassium, and vitamin D to the American diet. Turn to page 289 to learn more about this miraculous liquid.

> Switching from whole milk to skim milk can help you lose almost 7 pounds a year. According to the National Academy of Sciences, milk has ten times the bioavailability for calcium as spinach does!

Seventh: Spinach

Although spinach does contain oxalates that can bind calcium, a study in Japan found that young women who didn't get in daily intake of yellow and green vegetables, such spinach, had almost a fivefold risk of developing low bone mass, compared to those women who did. To learn more about this supernutritious green, see page 291.

TOP 7 SOURCES OF CHROMIUM

SNEAK-A-PEEK: RANKINGS AT A GLANCE

Unfortunately According to the National Institutes of Health, there is not a comprehensive data base on dietary chromium, because the chromium content of foods can be substantially affected by agricultural and manufacturing processes. However, many sources that discuss dietary chromium suggest that the following are some of the richest examples known.

Food	Amount
Brewer's yeast	1 tablespoon
Beer and red wine	12 ounces/5 ounces
Beef, organ, and processed meats	3 ounces
Aged cheese	1.5 ounces
Broccoli	1 cup
Mushrooms	1 cup
Grape juice	1 cup

Honorable mentions: Romaine lettuce, onions, oysters, whole grains, wheat germ, apple skins, potatoes, oats, prunes, nuts, asparagus

Best food groups: Meat, cheese, whole wheat products

What is chromium and why is it so important? Chromium is an essential mineral with a fundamental role in maintaining blood sugar levels. We only need very small amounts—that is why it is referred to as a "trace" mineral. It is part of the glucose tolerance factor (GTF), which helps increase the action of insulin in the body so glucose can be utilized more effectively. Chromium also helps activate various enzymes throughout the digestion process so our body can obtain energy from the different foods we eat.

Because chromium is needed in such slight amounts, deficiency is not seen often. In fact, chromium can also be absorbed through exposure to it in the environment. In certain cases, symptoms of chromium deficiency may include hyperinsulinemia, high blood pressure, high blood sugar levels, and insulin resistance.

HOW MUCH IS ENOUGH?

The DV for chromium is 80 mcg, based on a 2,000-calorie diet.

Dietary Reference Intakes (DRIs) for Chromium

Age	Children (mcg/day)	Males (mcg/day)	Females (mcg/day)	Pregnancy (mcg/day)	Lactation (mcg/day)
0–6 months	0.2				
7–12 months	5.5				
1–3 years	11				
4–8 years	15				
9–13 years		25	21		
14–18 years		35	24	29	44
19–50 years		35	25	30	45
51+ years		30	20		

SOURCE: Food and Nutrition Board, Institutes of Medicine, National Academies

Too much! Chromium toxicity due to food intake is very rare and hasn't been studied efficiently, no UL has been established. People with a history of liver and/or kidney problems should consult with their physician before taking any supplements that contain chromium.

Supplement it? Chromium is available in a variety of forms: chromium chloride, chromium picolinate, chromium polynicotinate, and chromium-enriched yeast. Which form is best has been the subject of much debate. Some studies have shown that chelated (meaning "clawed") forms of chromium, such as chromium picolinate and polynicotinate, where the chromium is bonded together with another substance, are better absorbed into the body. However, the chelating effect may also not allow enough of the chromium to be released in the body to be properly absorbed. Chromium in the polynicotinate form is often used to improve blood sugar control.

Brewer's Yeast

Brewer's yeast, also known as *Saccharomyces cerevisiae*, is actually a fungus used to make beer. It is sold as a powder of a tablet supplement and it is a rich source of B-complex vitamins, protein, and selenium. Other types of yeast, such as nutritional, baker's, and torula yeast, are actually low in chromium. In a study of fifty diabetic subjects, those who took brewer's yeast supplements for eight weeks had marked reductions in blood glucose, triglycerides, and LDL cholesterol levels, and elevated HDL cholesterol levels.

Beer and Red Wine

Studies have found that chromium can accrue during the fermentation process in some alcoholic beverages. A French study found that red wines varied in their chromium content anywhere from 7 to 90 mcg per liter. Syrah and Grenache varietals were the highest. So, that glass of wine or a can of beer may be providing your body with chromium, and you didn't even know it! Exciting news, but don't chug the whole bottle of wine or down a six-pack! Keep alcohol consumption moderate—one to two drinks per day for guys and one drink per day for women, per the American Heart Association.

Beef, Organ, and Processed Meats

Beef is an excellent source of chromium, protein, selenium, and zinc, and a good source of iron, niacin, riboflavin, and vitamin B_6. Elevated cholesterol, LDL cholesterol, and triglycerides can be complications of metabolic syndrome and diabetes. But when moderate amounts of lean beef were part of a DASH-style diet (see page 171), lipids were managed well as long as saturated fat was less than 7 percent.

Aged Cheese

True, some varieties of cheese are high in fat, but many are not—so you don't have to eliminate cheese from your diet if you are trying to watch your waistline! After all, just 1.5 ounces of aged cheese counts as a dairy serving, providing bone-building calcium and protein. Chromium has been found to help regulate blood sugar. The addition of dairy products, such as cheese, to the diet was found to lower the risk of metabolic syndrome, in turn benefiting blood pressure, cholesterol, and blood glucose levels.

Broccoli

Broccoli is one of the richest sources of chromium in the diet besides being loaded with other vitamins and minerals (see page 286). Broccoli is a great example of a low-calorie and nutrient-rich vegetable that aids in weight management and may play a role in managing blood glucose.

> California produces almost all the broccoli that is eaten in the United States; Americans eat, on average, 4 pounds per year. Consumption of this tasty vegetable has increased over 900 percent in the last twenty-five years.

Mushrooms

To learn more about the marvels of mushrooms, see page 289. Mushrooms are also rich in substances called beta-glucans which possess immune-stimulating and cholesterol-lowering benefits. Beta-glucans are highest in the oyster, shiitake, and split gill mushroom varieties. Mushrooms may be a worthy opponent in the fight against dia-besity. Research has shown that swapping out high-calorie, dense foods for low-calorie yet filling foods such as mushrooms can help aid in managing weight yet feeling satisfied after meals. Reducing weight can help reduce the risk of type 2 diabetes.

Grape Juice

Not surprising to find that grape juice is a good source of chromium, in light of wine's being a great source, too! Grape juice is an excellent source of manganese, powerful antioxidants called polyphenols, and vitamin C. I don't know about you but I've always found grape juice to be pretty sweet and assumed that it raises blood glucose quickly. But in a study of sixty-four healthy individuals, average blood glucose dropped instead of rising after drinking grape juice. Go figure!

TOP 7 SOURCES OF COPPER

SNEAK-A-PEEK: RANKINGS AT A GLANCE

Ranking	Food	Serving	Amount (mcg)
First Place	**Beef liver (cooked)**	**3 ounces**	**12,400**
First Runner-Up	**Pacific/Eastern oysters (raw)**	**3 ounces**	**12,000**
Second Runner-Up	**Lobster (cooked)**	**3 ounces**	**1,550**
Fourth	Shiitake mushrooms	1 cup	1,299
Fifth	King crab (cooked)	3 ounces	1,055
Sixth	Baking chocolate	1 ounce	917
Seventh	White mushrooms (cooked)	1 cup	786

SOURCE: USDA National Nutrient Database for Standard Reference, Release 24

Honorable mentions: Sunflower seeds, cocoa powder, soybeans, cashews, white beans

Best food groups: Seafood, meat, nuts, legumes, vegetables

What is copper and why is it so important? Your body only needs just a smidge of copper, but that little amount is vital to support necessary functions, such as hemoglobin's ability to absorb iron and carry oxygen via the red blood cells throughout the body. Copper also plays a role in supporting normal growth and a healthy immune system. Deficiencies are rare, but signs can include anemia, infertility, joint problems, osteoporosis, abnormal cholesterol levels, and poor immune function.

Did you know? Wearing copper bracelets or taking copper supplements were once thought of as being curative for arthritis. No solid research exists to support that claim. However, you can derive copper from drinking out of copper goblets, drinking and cooking with water that passes through copper pipes, and using all-copper cookware.

HOW MUCH IS ENOUGH?

The DV for copper is 2 mg, based on a 2,000-calorie diet.

Dietary Reference Intakes (DRIs) for Copper

Age	Children (mcg/day)	Males (mcg/day)	Females (mcg/day)	Pregnancy (mcg/day)	Lactation (mcg/day)
0–6 months	200				
6–12 months	200				
1–3 years	340				
4–8 years	440				
9–13 years		700	700		
14–18 years		890	890	1,000	1,300
19–50 years		900	900	1,000	1,300
51+ years		900	900		

SOURCE: Food and Nutrition Board, Institutes of Medicine, National Academies

Too much! Although, copper toxicity is rare, a UL has been set at 10,000 mcg (10 mg) for adults. Studies have found that acute copper toxicity causes a number of problems, including but not limited to abdominal pain, nausea/vomiting, diarrhea, jaundice, headache, and weakness.

Supplement it? Most multivitamins include copper as part of the featured minerals. Copper is also available as a separate oral supplement. Taking too much copper has been linked to vomiting and even death. Those diagnosed with Wilson's disease, which can cause copper buildup in the body, are advised to avoid supplements with copper in them.

First Place: Beef Liver

Read all about the benefits of beef liver on page 286. In the battle of obesity, many have turned to bariatric surgery (where the size of the stomach is surgically reduced). Although this can be an effective tool in weight loss, it is not without concerns, especially due to increased deficiencies of nutrients, such as copper, postsurgery. Adding liver periodically to a bariatric diet may be beneficial in helping to overcome copper deficiencies. (If this applies to you, work with a bariatric dietitian to know when such foods as liver can be introduced.)

First Runner-Up: Pacific or Eastern Oysters

There are several different kinds of oysters, each having unique, distinct tastes. Depending on the soil, location, and climate of where the oysters were harvested, the flavor can range from salty to sweet, with different undertones like herbs or butter. Oysters are micronutrient powerhouses; just one half-shell supplies almost all or all of the daily needs for copper, iron, magnesium, and vitamin B_{12}. (See page 289 for more about oysters.) A study has shown that oysters had a better lipid-lowering effect than did soybean protein when added to the diet of rats.

Hard shell vs. soft shell? Lobsters usually shed their shells three or four times a year, until they are about seven years old. While they are waiting for their hard shell to develop, they can be classified as "soft-shell" lobsters—both varieties taste great!

Second Runner-Up: Lobster

Besides being an excellent source of copper, lobster is also a source of vanadium, which may benefit the management of diabetes (of course, without all that drawn butter on it!). It is also rich in other nutrients; see page 289. Each

3-ounce serving only has about 60 mg of cholesterol, which is well below the daily recommendation of 300 mg per day.

Fourth: Shiitake Mushrooms

The shiitake mushroom is now the second most widely produced mushroom in the world. See page 289 to learn more about this mushroom's benefits.

Fifth: King Crab

Crabs, and king crabs in particular, are an excellent source of copper, in addition to the numerous nutrients listed on page 287. In a small study of eighteen men, crab was one of four shellfish found helpful in lowering triglycerides and cholesterol.

Sixth: Baking Chocolate

Baking chocolate is used primarily as an ingredient in recipes for brownies, cakes, and frostings. It is also known as bitter or unsweetened chocolate, and contains 100% cacao. Unsweetened baking chocolate should contain between 50 and 58 percent cocoa butter. Cocoa contains a variety of vitamins and minerals and plant antioxidants known as flavanols, and may be one of the most antioxidant-rich foods known.

On the one hand, literally, turning to chocolate to ease your pain may not be the best idea. A study of twenty-four men found that sugar acted like an analgesic when they consumed it while holding on to extremely cold bars. They were able to hold on longer with the sugar solution alone. But when cocoa was added to it, their pain tolerance decreased by 30 percent! However, over 250 intervention studies in the last ten years, plus ten review and meta-analysis' studies, have shown that the benefits of eating chocolate far outweigh this unique negative. Cocoa polyphenols found in baking chocolate raise nitric oxide, which promotes vasodilation, decreases inflammation and the stickiness of blood cells, boosts our antioxidant system and insulin sensitivity, and reduces blood pressure and LDL cholesterol. Plus, research has also suggested that adding in flavanol-rich cocoa to our diet regularly helps reduce the risk of dying from most diseases!

Seventh: White Mushrooms

Read all about this nutrient-packed little button on page 289.

There are 14,000 known mushroom species; however, that's only a small percentage of the estimated 140,000 total varieties! Although some are poisonous to eat, there are more than enough of the kind to enjoy in salads and side dishes.

TOP 7 SOURCES OF IODINE

SNEAK-A-PEEK: RANKINGS AT A GLANCE

Ranking	Food	Serving	Amount (mcg)
First Place	Seaweed	1 gram	16–2,984
First Runner-Up	Cod (baked)	3 ounces	99
Second Runner-Up	Yogurt	1 cup	75
Fourth	Iodized salt	¼ teaspoon (1.5 grams)	71
Fifth	Milk	8 ounces	56
Sixth	Shrimp (cooked)	3 ounces	35
Seventh	Eggs (cooked)	1 large	24

Source: USDA National Nutrient Database for Standard Reference, Release 24

Honorable mentions: Chocolate ice cream, bread, fish sticks, tuna (canned in oil), prunes, Cheddar cheese, lima beans, apple juice

Best food groups: Seaweed, seafood, dairy

What is iodine and why is it so important? Iodine is an essential mineral that is required to make protein and enzymes for chemical reactions in the body. It is of particular importance in the thyroid gland as it is needed, along with the amino acid tyrosine, to create thyroid hormones that help regulate metabolism. Iodine is also essential to the skeletal and central nervous systems of developing fetuses. A lack of iodine in the human body causes the thyroid to overreact and swell up in an attempt to capture more iodine. This results in the swelling of the neck, commonly referred to as goiter. Back in the early twentieth century, most brands of salt began to add iodine to prevent the development of goiters, which were prevalent around the Great Lakes area of the United States.

HOW MUCH IS ENOUGH?

The DV for iodine is 150 mcg, based on a 2,000-calorie diet.

Dietary Reference Intakes (DRIs) for Iodine

Age	Children (mcg/day)	Males (mcg/day)	Females (mcg/day)	Pregnancy (mcg/day)	Lactation (mcg/day)
0–6 months	110				
7–12 months	130				
1–3 years	90				
4–8 years	90				
9–13 years		120	120		
14–18 years		150 (900 UL)	150 (900 UL)	220	290
19+ years		150 (1,100 UL)	150 (1,100 UL)	220	290

SOURCE: Food and Nutrition Board, Institutes of Medicine, National Academies

Too much! Typically, food does not contain high enough doses of iodine to have harmful effects; rather, iodine overload comes from chemical exposure. Ironically, high intakes of iodine can cause the same symptoms as a deficiency, namely goiters and hypothyroidism. Excess iodine can stimulate thyroid stimulating hormone (TSH), which can produce a goiter, and excess intakes can also lead to thyroiditis and potentially thyroid papillary cancer.

Did you know? According to the CDC, tincture of iodine (often in the form of inedible povidone-iodine, such as Betadine) is used in presurgical procedures to kill and also prevent microorganisms from growing. It is quite effective in reducing infection rate and increasing wound healing. In chemistry, iodine gas is thought of as being violent. Our mineral name *iodine* is derived from the term *iodes*, the Greek word for "violent."

Supplement it? Most multivitamins contain iodine but you may purchase them without it, as some people have allergic reactions to iodine or may be on iodine therapy. Vegans may be at risk for low iodine intake, so vegan women of child-bearing age should supplement with 150 mcg of iodine daily.

First Place: Seaweed

Kombu is known as "the king of seaweeds" and is one of the richest sources of iodine of all of the sea vegetables. It is an essential staple in the Japanese diet and is used to make dashi (stock); it has a wonderful umami taste. It can also be rehydrated or chopped up and added to stews, soups, and casseroles. A strip of it added to a pot of beans, while cooking, reduces the gas-producing carbohydrate called raffinose. Kombu and other brown algae are potent sources of a carbohydrate called fucoidan that possesses anti-inflammatory, antioxidant, and anticancer properties. Fucoidan has been shown to kill human stomach and colon cancer cells, battle immune-related diseases, and keep tumor growth at bay.

First Runner-Up: Cod

Cod is a white, mild-flavored fish that flakes when eaten. In England, cod is the most common fish ingredient in that nation's staple dish, fish and chips. Cod typically weighs between 10 and 25 pounds, but some have been caught as large as 220 pounds. Cod liver oil is an important source of omega-3 fatty acids and vitamins A, D, and E. The fish is an excellent source of iodine and selenium, and a great source of magnesium, niacin, phosphorus, and vitamins B_6 and B_{12}. Like chicken and turkey, cod is also an abundant source of the amino acid tryptophan, which has been associated with increased sleepiness. Eating cod, or any fish that is either broiled or baked instead of fried, can help reduce a person's risk of atrial fibrillation, the most common form of heart arrhythmia. Those older adults who had higher plasma levels of omega-3 fats from food sources such as cod were less likely to experience atrial fibrillation later on in life.

Second Runner-Up: Yogurt

Get the skinny on low-fat plain yogurt on page 292. Boston University researchers found that those subjects who reported eating yogurt and salty fish had the highest level of urinary iodine, compared to those who didn't eat those items regularly.

Fourth: Iodized Salt

Until the 1920s, iodine deficiency was prevalent in the Great Lakes, Appalachian, and Northwestern regions of the United States. Salt was then required to be iodized and shortly afterward, goiters in the United States decreased substantially. Researchers have found wide variation in the iodine content in common foods as well as iodized salt products. Almost 70 percent of all sodium consumed in the United States comes from processed foods; however, producers of commercially prepared food are not required by law to use iodized salt. There is also concern that a call for decreased sodium may also decrease iodine in the diet, so it may be to our best interest to require the use of iodized salt in processed food. Since the 1970s, urinary iodine levels have decreased by nearly 50 percent but average levels still remain in the sufficient range. CDC researchers found that many women are only borderline sufficient in iodine. This may have to do with their not consuming adequate amounts of iodine-rich foods, such as sea vegetables and fish, dairy, and iodized salt.

Fifth: Milk

Read all about the virtues of 2% milk on page 289. Back in 2004, a sampling of eighteen different brands of cow's milk in the Boston area revealed that 1-cup samples varied greatly, containing 88 to 168 mcg of iodine per serving.

Sixth: Shrimp

These tasty crustaceans are swimmers, rather than crawlers like their counterparts lobster and crayfish. They are also low in calories and saturated fat, making them a great alternative protein source for more fatty meats. Shrimp are an excellent source of iodine, phosphorus, selenium, and vitamin B_{12}, and also a good source of copper, niacin, vitamin B_6, and zinc.

Shrimp are high in cholesterol. But in a peer-reviewed study, researchers found that adding 300 grams (10.5 ounces) of shrimp to the diet per day showed a decreased ratio of total cholesterol to HDL cholesterol. Additionally, the group that ate shrimp lowered their triglycerides by 13 percent!

Seventh: Eggs

Eggs are a great affordable source of high-quality protein. One large egg provides 6.3 g of protein for only 72 calories. Eggs are also vital to food chemistry. We use them for browning, coagulation, emulsification, and foaming of many foods. See page 287 for the other nutritional benefits of eggs. Adding iodine to the feed of chickens via natural sources such as sea kelp or iodine-rich yeast has been found to triple the amount of iodine normally available in the egg. Unfortunately, this is not common practice, commercially . . . yet!

TOP 7 SOURCES OF IRON

SNEAK-A-PEEK: RANKINGS AT A GLANCE

Ranking	Food	Serving	Amount (mg)
First Place	Liver* (pork, chicken, or beef, cooked)	3 ounces	5.24–9.5
First Runner-Up	Soybeans (cooked)	1 cup	8.8
Second Runner-Up	White beans (cooked)	1 cup	7.83
Fourth	Lentils (cooked)	1 cup	6.6
Fifth	Spinach (cooked)	1 cup	6.43
Sixth	Kidney beans (cooked)	1 cup	5.2
Seventh	Jerusalem artichokes	1 cup	5.1

*Asterisked food contains heme iron. Plant substances such as polyphenols, phytate, calcium, and myricetin have been shown to reduce nonheme bioavailability.
SOURCE: USDA National Nutrient Database for Standard Reference, Release 24

Heme honorable mentions: Beef chuck, clams, turkey (dark and light meat), chicken leg, bluefin tuna, chicken breast, halibut, crab. pork, white tuna (canned)

Non-heme honorable mentions: Fortified cereals, long-grain enriched rice, lima beans. navy beans, firm tofu, black and pinto beans, molasses. Adding ascorbic acid (vitamin C), meat, and alcohol can increase iron availability from non-heme sources.

Best food groups: Meat, seafood, beans

What is iron and why is it so important? Iron is one of the most abundant minerals on Earth and is vital to our existence, yet the World Health Organization deems iron deficiency the number one nutritional disorder that plagues our world. Iron is a mineral whose job is to bind oxygen in red blood cells. Without it, our red blood cells would not be able to carry oxygen for our body to function! This mineral controls fifty genes, and maybe even more, directly or indirectly. The intestine decides how much iron is absorbed at any given moment, based on need.

We lose about half of our daily iron loss from our intestine, and the other half from shedding skin cells and urine. Main reasons for iron deficiency are: low intake of bioavailable iron (American vegetarians can have diets that contain 10 percent bioavailable iron, and therefore require 1.8 times more iron consumption than those eating a mixed diet containing meat); inadequate absorption; decreased stomach acidity, commonly caused by the bacteria *H. pylori*; and excessive blood loss. Symptoms of mild to moderate forms of iron deficiencies include impaired cognitive function, decreased immunity, fatigue, inability to regulate body temperature properly, shortened gestation in pregnancy, preterm birth, and lower birth weight.

HOW MUCH IS ENOUGH?

The DV for iron is 18 mg, based on a 2,000-calorie diet.

Dietary Reference Intakes (DRIs) for Iron

Age	Children (mg/day)	Males (mg/day)	Females (mg/day)	Pregnancy (mg/day)	Lactation (mg/day)
0–6 months	0.27				
7–12 months	11				
1–3 years	7				
4–8 years	10				
9–13 years		8	8		
14–18 years		11	15	27	10
19–50 years		8	18	27	9
51+ years		8	8		

SOURCE: Food and Nutrition Board, Institutes of Medicine, National Academies

Too much! Some suffer from blood disorders that cause iron to build up in the body. High iron is a leading risk factor for heart disease in post-menopausal women and men. One of the most effective ways of decreasing iron stores is to donate blood. In fact, donating a pint of blood removes about 200 to 250 mg of iron from the bloodstream and can reduce a person's risk for heart disease.

Did you know? Women using contraceptives lose on average 60 percent less blood during menses. Their need for iron is reduced to 11 mg per day, compared to 18 mg per day for women who do not use oral contraceptives. Those who run regularly may also require as much as 30 percent more iron, due to ruptured blood cells in their feet!

Supplement it? There are two forms of supplemental iron: ferrous and ferric. The best absorbable forms of iron are ferrous fumarate, ferrous sulfate, and ferrous gluconate, the best of the three being ferrous fumarate, because it has higher percentage of elemental iron. Men and postmenopausal women should avoid supplements with iron unless advised by a physician.

Shocker Food!

Want your children to perform better in school? You might want to consider giving them braunschweiger, or any other food high in iron, for breakfast. Iron deficiency is the most common nutrient deficiency in the United Stated and it has been related to poor cognitive development, intellectual performance, and academic achievement. Good news is that correcting iron deficiency can help kids do better in both mental and physical performance. See page 290 for more about this nutritious liver-based sausage.

First Place: Liver (pork, chicken, or beef)

See pages 286 and 287 to learn more about liver. Chicken liver contains the most heme, which makes it the most bioavailable form of iron of any food!

First Runner-Up: Soybeans

Soy, because of the plant compound called phytate, has mostly been considered a less than optimal source of iron. However, all soy may not be created equal. A Japanese study found that when a fermented soybean liquid called shoyu (a.k.a. soy sauce) was added to the diet, iron absorption was enhanced in both animal and human studies. Turn to page 291 for the other benefits of soy.

Second Runner-Up: White Beans

White beans are an excellent source of copper, folate, iron, magnesium, manganese, and phosphorus, and a good source of calcium, potassium, and zinc. White beans have also been shown to lower LDL cholesterol levels.

Fourth: Lentils

Available in varieties ranging in color from yellow to red-orange to green, lentils are an excellent source iron as well as numerous other minerals and vitamins (see page 289). The latest dietary guidelines suggest that Americans fill half their plate with fruits and vegetables to meet the recommended serving amounts of produce. The good news is that legumes, such as lentils, count as a vegetable. A Penn State study found that though lentils and other legumes provide an array of nutrients that could mitigate disease and improve health, on any given day only 7.9 percent of adults consume legumes.

Fifth: Spinach

Spinach is an excellent source of iron as well as a slew of other nutrients (see page 291). Although spinach contains nonheme iron and the oxalate component is thought to decrease iron absorption, a human study found very little influence of oxalates in the absorption and bioavailability of this mineral.

Sixth: Kidney Beans

Kidney beans are an excellent source of fiber, manganese, molybdenum, potassium, phosphorus, and protein, and a good source of copper and magnesium. They are an excellent source of folate and a good source of thiamine and vitamin K. Although kidney beans are a rich source of iron, they are also high in phytates and polyphenols, which can block iron absorption. White beans may be a good companion to mix with kidney beans, as they were found to contain an unknown substance that increases iron bioavailability.

> Kidney beans are thought to have originated in Peru and Indian traders brought them throughout South and Central America. The red bean made its way to Europe on the mid-fifteenth century and was brought to North America via exploring Spanish conquistadors.

Seventh: Jerusalem Artichokes

Jerusalem artichokes are technically tubers that are similar to potatoes, but their carbohydrate content is mainly made up of inulin rather than starch. Inulin has prebiotic properties that help friendly bacteria thrive. Besides

> Jeruselum artichokes are not from Jerusalem or anywhere near the Middle East. In fact, they hail from regions of North America and were brought to France by early settlers.

being a excellent source of iron, Jerusalem artichokes are also a good source of fiber, phosphorus, and potassium.

TOP 7 SOURCES OF MAGNESIUM

SNEAK-A-PEEK: RANKINGS AT A GLANCE

Ranking	Food	Serving	Amount (mcg)
First Place	Spinach (cooked)	1 cup	163
First Runner-Up	Pumpkin seeds	1 ounce	156
Second Runner-Up	Soybeans	1 cup	148
Fourth	White beans (cooked)	1 cup	134
Fifth	Black beans (cooked)	1 cup	120
Sixth	Brazil nuts	1 ounce	107
Seventh	Lima beans (cooked)	1 cup	101

SOURCE: USDA National Nutrient Database for Standard Reference, Release 24

Honorable mentions: Beet greens, navy beans, cowpeas, great northern beans, tomato paste, trail mix, cooked oat bran

Best food groups: Beans, nuts, dark green vegetables, poultry, lean meat, unrefined grains

What is magnesium and why is it so important? Magnesium is responsible for over three hundred biochemical reactions in the body including maintaining normal muscle and nerve function, keeping heart rhythm steady, supporting a healthy immune system, and keeping bones strong to prevent breaks or fractures. Magnesium has also been shown to help regulate blood sugar levels and blood pressure.

Magnesium deficiency in the United Sates is rare but can be caused by inadequate intake, as well as digestive health challenges. Inflammatory bowel disease such as Crohn's disease can cause decreased absorption of a variety of nutrients, including magnesium. Vomiting or diarrhea can cause a deficiency in magnesium as well. Early signs of magnesium deficiency include loss of appetite, nausea and vomiting, fatigue and weakness, numbness and tingling, muscle contractions and cramps, seizures, personality changes, abnormal heart rhythms, and coronary spasms.

Did you know? Poorly controlled diabetes may increase the need for magnesium due to increased nutrient loss in the urine. The elderly are at most risk for magnesium deficiency, according to NHANES, because they consume fewer calories, compared to younger populations. Additionally, certain medications, such as diuretics, can lead to excessive magnesium loss.

HOW MUCH IS ENOUGH?

The DV for magnesium is 400 mg, based on a 2,000-calorie diet.

Dietary Reference Intakes (DRIs) for Magnesium

Age (years)	Children (mg/day)	Males (mg/day)	Females (mg/day)	Pregnancy (mg/day)	Lactation (mg/day)
0–6 months	30				
7–12 months	75				
1–3 years	80				
4–8 years	130				
9–13 years		240	240		
14–18 years		410	360	400	360
19–30 years		400	310	350	310
31+ years		420	320	360	320

SOURCE: Food and Nutrition Board, Institutes of Medicine, National Academies

Too much! Use of over-the-counter supplements and drugs containing magnesium has become more prevalent over the years. Antacids, laxatives, multivitamins, and even relaxation tinctures can contain magnesium. The first sign that you've ingested too much magnesium is usually diarrhea. Other symptoms can include generalized weakness (both in muscle and in bones), sleepiness, very low blood pressure, and shortness of breath.

Supplement it? You can find magnesium in multivitamins and bone-building compounds, and as individual supplements in the form of magnesium oxide, magnesium sulfate, and magnesium carbonate. In a study that compared magnesium supplements, magnesium chloride and magnesium lactate had the highest bioavailability.

First Place: Spinach

We've all had drilled through our heads that fresh is best and canned foods are nutritionally void. *Not true!* Go figure that cooked and canned spinach, not raw, ranked the highest magnesium food on this list! See page 291 for the many other nutrients in this power-packed leafy green vegetable. An animal study showed that cooked spinach still contains oxalate, which is believed to inhibit the bioavailability of magnesium. However, the study showed that magnesium absorption was not impaired.

First Runner-Up: Pumpkin Seeds

Magnesium-rich pumpkin and other squash seeds are among the healthiest seeds in the world, especially for men, because their nutritional profile (see page 290) benefits prostate health. They

> Pumpkin seeds found in Mexico date back over 7,500 years. This seed played a large role in Native American cuisine and medicine.

are also a great source of beta-sitosterol, a plant sterol that helps lower cholesterol and reduce the swelling of the prostate.

Second Runner-Up: Soybeans

Soybeans are sold in various forms, including as fresh or frozen edamame, fresh mature soybeans, and dried soybeans. *Edamame* refers to the raw immature soybean that varies in nutritional content from the mature version. Soy is an excellent source of magnesium, in addition to being a complete source of protein, meaning it has all of the essential amino acids that humans must consume in order to remain healthy. Soybeans have been studied among large populations for many years and offer some promise for reducing the risk of developing breast, prostate, ovarian, and uterine cancer. See page 291 to read more about this remarkable legume.

Fourth: White Beans

See page 286 to learn more about white beans. You may know this legume as the Boston bean, white coco bean, pea bean, *alubia chica,* haricot, or navy bean (see page 286).

Fifth: Black Beans

Black beans are loaded with prebiotics (nutrients for bacteria) to allow healthy bacteria (probiotics) to flourish. Besides being an excellent source of magnesium and other nutrients (see page 286), black beans are rich in soluble fiber and higher in polyphenols than lentils and chickpeas.

This may be the most popular bean in the western hemisphere. It is used in many popular dishes, including in Brazil, in *feijoada*; in Venezuela, as part of *pabellón criollo*; and in the United States in the Mexican-American black bean burrito.

Sixth: Brazil Nuts

In addition to being a terrific source of magnesium, Brazil nuts are an excellent source of copper, phosphorus, and selenium, and a good source of fiber, manganese, and thiamine. A 1999–2004 NHANES study found those who consumed trees nuts, such as Brazil nuts, had a higher increase in average magnesium and overall diet quality and lower sodium intake compared to those who did not.

Brazil nut trees are native to the Amazon rainforest and other regions located throughout South America. The Spanish introduced Brazil nuts to Europe in the 1500s, where they were referred to as *almendras de los Andes* (almonds of the Andes). Bolivia, Brazil, and Peru are presently the chief producing countries.

Seventh: Lima Beans

Besides being a great source of magnesium, lima beans have a slew of other nutrients (see page 286). Baked and lima
beans were found to be the most effective
varieties of beans to lower cholesterol in an
animal study.

> Lima beans are native to
> Central America and are
> thought to have begun
> being cultivated over
> seven thousand years ago.

TOP 7 SOURCES OF MANGANESE

SNEAK-A-PEEK: RANKINGS AT A GLANCE

Ranking	Food	Serving	Amount (mg)
First Place	**Teff (cooked)**	**½ cup**	**3.6**
First Runner-Up	**Pineapple**	**1 cup**	**2.79**
Second Runner-Up	**Pine nuts**	**1 ounce**	**2.49**
Fourth	Chickpeas (cooked)	1 cup	1.93
Fifth	Hazelnuts	1 ounce	1.75
Sixth	Spinach (cooked)	1 cup	1.68
Seventh	Raspberries	1 cup	1.62

SOURCE: USDA National Nutrient Database for Standard Reference, Release 24

Honorable mentions: Okra, oat bran, bulgur, barley, coconut

Best food groups: Fortified cereals, whole grains, nuts, legumes, seeds, tea,
leafy green vegetables

What is manganese and why is it so important? Manganese is an essential
trace element in human body. Many enzymes depend on manganese to
create metalloenzymes, which play a role in the utilization of glucose and
the breaking down of proteins and fats. It is stored mostly in bones, but
you can also see a good amount stored in the kidney and liver. Maintaining a balanced diet high in fruits, vegetables, nuts, and whole grains is the
best dietary approach to getting in enough manganese.

Deficiencies include ataxia (lack of coordination), fainting, hearing loss, weak tendons and ligaments, impaired glucose metabolism and reduced insulin production, myasthenia gravis (loss of muscle strength), infertility, diseases of the skeletal structure, impaired growth, elevated blood pressure, atherosclerosis, poor immune function, and selenium deficiency.

HOW MUCH IS ENOUGH?

The DV for manganese is 2 mg, based on a 2,000-calorie diet.

Dietary Reference Intakes (DRIs) for Manganese

Age	Children (mg/day)	Males (mg/day)	Females (mg/day)	Pregnancy (mg/day)	Lactation (mg/day)
0–6 months	0.003				
7–12 months	0.6				
1–3 years	1.2				
4–8 years	1.5				
9–13 years		1.9	1.6		
14–18 years		2.2	1.6	2.0	2.6
19+ years		2.3	1.8	2.0	2.6

SOURCE: Food and Nutrition Board, Institutes of Medicine, National Academies

Too much! When we ingest too much manganese, our body attempts to reduce the amount that is absorbed to protect against toxicity by combining manganese with other minerals, such as calcium and iron. Excess manganese decreases the ability to absorb iron. Iron deficiencies typically only occur if there is long-term exposure to high levels of manganese, but this is rare in a typical American diet and is usually the result of industrial pollution. Symptoms of toxicity are hypertension and Parkinson's-like signs and symptoms.

Did you know? Manganese is a key ingredient in the steel-making process and is responsible for prevention of oxidation or rust. Not surprisingly, manganese functions much the same way in the body, as an antioxidant preventing free radical damage to cells and DNA.

Supplement it? Manganese is typically found in multivitamins and bone support formulations. However, it can be purchased as a single ingredient. Supplementing manganese can impact iron absorption. Manganese sulfate is the most common form, found in dietary supplements, but other forms are available.

First Place: Teff

Teff holds the title of "smallest grain in the world." In fact, it is so small that it was given the Amharic name *teffa*, which means "lost"—which would most certainly be the case if you were unfortunate to drop a kernel on the ground! When it comes to nutrition, teff is no lightweight, and in fact, besides being the best source of manganese, is an excellent source of copper and a good source of fiber, iron, magnesium, phosphorus, protein, thiamine, vitamin B$_6$, and zinc. Teff has over twice the iron of other grains, and three times the calcium (though it is not considered a "good" source of calcium).

> Teff provides the main source of nutrition to over two-thirds of Ethiopians mainly in the form of a flatbread they enjoy called *injera*.

First Runner-Up: Pineapple

Canned pineapple (the kind packed in juice) could be yet another shiny example of a shocker food, as it is the second-richest source of manganese and also an excellent source of vitamin C. Pineapple is also rich in an enzyme called bromelain, which has powerful anti-inflammatory properties. An animal study found mice that were fed pineapple juice had markedly reduced inflammation of tissues associated with colitis. However, to obtain this enzyme, fresh pineapple has more bromelain than canned.

Second Runner-Up: Pine Nuts

Tree nuts, such as manganese-rich pine nuts, contribute significantly to overall nutrition in those cultures that consume them regularly.

So here's a real shocker, though: It might not be worth your while to depend on pine nuts with any regularity for your daily quota of manganese, or any other nutrient, for that matter. More and more cases of "pine mouth" and allergic reactions have been reported after ingesting pine nuts. Apparently, there is a substance that causes a bitter taste in the mouth after ingesting. Occasional use is probably not a worry, but certainly contact your doctor if you experience swelling or a continued bitter taste in your mouth.

> Pine nuts are found within pinecones, but don't eat the kind you may find in your backyard. There are two main species on the market: the Mediterranean or Italian pine nut and the stronger-flavored Chinese variety. The Roman Legions carried pine kernels during their long marches on their quest for dominance.

Fourth: Chickpeas

Manganese-rich chickpeas are a wonderful source of other minerals; see page 287). A study that looked at a variety of legumes found that chickpeas and lentils had the greatest effect on lowering blood glucose after a meal.

Fifth: Hazelnuts

The terms filbert and hazelnut are often used interchangeably as they refer to the same nut. Besides being an excellent source of manganese, hazelnuts are a hotbed of other vitamins and minerals; see page 288. They are also rich in plant polyphenols, which are mainly found in the outer skin of the nut. Roasting was found to dramatically reduce polyphenols, mainly because the skin was reduced or eliminated in the roasting process.

Sixth: Spinach

Manganese-rich foods like spinach may be helpful in reversing symptoms of deficiencies such as weak muscles. For the many other benefits of this superhealthy veggie, turn to page 291.

Seventh: Raspberries

Raspberries are an excellent source of vitamin C and fiber and a good source of vitamin K. Besides being loaded with manganese, raspberries are also high anthocyanins and ellagitannins, antioxidant-rich plant nutrients that may play a role in fighting a host of diseases, including cancer.

TOP 7 SOURCES OF MOLYBDENUM

SNEAK-A-PEEK: RANKINGS AT A GLANCE

Ranking	Food	Serving	Amount (mcg)
First Place	Navy beans (cooked)	1 cup	196
First Runner-Up	Cowpeas (cooked)	1 cup	180
Second Runner-Up	Yellow split peas (cooked)	1 cup	149
Fourth	Lentils (cooked)	1 cup	148
Fifth	Lima beans (cooked)	1 cup	142
Sixth	Kidney beans (cooked)	1 cup	132
Seventh	Black beans (cooked)	1 cup	130

SOURCE: USDA National Nutrient Database for Standard Reference, Release 24

Honorable mentions: Almonds, oats, peanuts, yogurt, potatoes, bread, green split peas, dark greens

Best food groups: Legumes, nuts, whole grains

What is molybdenum and why is it so important? Similar to other trace minerals, molybdenum is only needed in small amounts but is crucial for enzymatic reactions that occur in the body. The active form, called molybdenum cofactor, is needed for helping to eliminate toxic substances. One toxic waste product that molybdenum helps get rid of is purines, which can increase uric acid in the body—especially in those who have gouty arthritis.

Typically, deficiencies are not seen in the healthy population. The only cases that have been studied have occurred in hospitals, and in those with inborn errors of metabolism or who have been on total parenteral nutrition (TPN). Some of the symptoms include tachycardia, headache, and coma.

As part of its detoxification role, molybdenum helps neutralize nitrosamines, which have been linked to cancer development, and it also helps rid the body of excessive copper, which occurs in metabolic diseases, such as Wilson's disease.

HOW MUCH IS ENOUGH?

The DV is for molybdenum is 75 mcg, based on a 2,000-calorie diet.

Dietary Reference Intakes (DRIs) for Molybdenum

Age	Children (mcg/day)	Males (mcg/day)	Females (mcg/day)	Pregnancy (mcg/day)	Lactation (mcg/day)
0–6 months	2				
6–12 months	3				
1–3 years	17				
4–8 years	22				
9–13 years		34	34		
14–18 years		43	43	50	50
19–50 years		45	45	50	50
51+ years		45	45		

SOURCE: Food and Nutrition Board, Institutes of Medicine, National Academies

Too much! The UL for this mineral has been set at 2,000 mcg per day. However, molybdenum being a trace mineral means toxicity is rare in healthy humans. Toxicity from supplements has been reported, where the symptoms included acute psychosis, seizures, and various neurological issues.

Supplement it? As mentioned earlier, molybdenum deficiencies are rarely seen in humans, therefore supplementation is also rarely needed.

First Place: Navy Beans

See page 286 for the many other benefits of this nutritious bean. In addition to supplying molybdenum, navy beans are also rich in a group of plant nutrients called saponins, which studies show help lower harmful

Shocker Food! ────────────────────

Molybdenum isn't found in many animal products, but cottage cheese is an excellent source of the nutrient. One cup has 20 mcg of molybdenum though significantly less than beans! Read more about cottage cheese on page 287.

fats in the blood that lead to heart disease and also lower cancer risk and blood glucose response. Saponins have also been found to reduce cavities and may work as an antidote against acute lead poisoning.

First Runner-Up: Cowpeas

Go to page 287 to read more about this legume, also known as black-eyed peas. According to the Academy of Nutrition and Dietetics, including high-fiber foods, such as cowpeas that have both soluble and insoluble dietary fibers, can help manage cholesterol, blood glucose, and insulin levels while promoting normal bowel regularity, and help prevent the development of diverticular disease.

Second Runner-Up: Yellow Split Peas

Split peas are also an excellent source of folate iron, manganese, molybdenum, pantothenic acid, phosphorus, and thiamine, and are also a good source of choline, magnesium, niacin, potassium, and zinc. Men and women who were fed a diet that included yellow pea flour that equaled ½ cup of peas daily had reduced insulin and insulin resistance.

Fourth: Lentils

Learn all about this power-packed little bean on page 289. Most of the fiber in lentils is soluble, the kind that helps lower cholesterol and prevent spikes in blood sugar. In the famous Harvard Nurses' Health Study involving over ninety thousand women, it was found that those women who ate more legumes (such as lentils) were less likely to develop breast cancer.

Fifth: Lima Beans

Besides containing molybdenum, lima beans are an excellent source of copper, fiber, folate, iron, magnesium, manganese, potassium, protein, and thiamine. Lima beans are rich in the plant nutrients coumestrol and saponin, which research suggests may help fight cancer and lower cholesterol.

Sixth: Kidney Beans

Kidney beans are an excellent source of folate, iron, manganese, molybdenum, phosphorus, and potassium, and a good source of the magnesium, thiamine, and vitamin K. Red kidney beans rank right behind black beans as the second highest in antioxidants and are an excellent choice at a salad bar. Those who are sensitive to the sulfates added to many food items at salad bars are often low in molybdenum, whose job is to detox the body of such compounds.

Seventh: Black Beans

Black beans are loaded with prebiotics (nutrients for bacteria) to allow healthy bacteria (probiotics) to flourish. Besides black beans' being an excellent source of molybdenum, Michigan State researchers found when testing for antioxidant capacity that black beans were the highest of any bean, followed by red, brown, yellow, and lastly white beans. To read more about this supernutritious bean, turn to page 286.

TOP 7 SOURCES OF PHOSPHORUS

SNEAK-A-PEEK: RANKINGS AT A GLANCE

Ranking	Food	Serving	Amount (mg)
First Place	Ricotta cheese	1 cup	450
First Runner-Up	Soybeans (cooked)	1 cup	421
Second Runner-Up	Sardines (canned)	3 ounces	417

continues

continued

Ranking	Food	Serving	Amount (mg)
Fourth	Beef liver (cooked)	3 ounces	412
Fifth	Lentils (cooked)	1 cup	356
Sixth	Yogurt	1 cup	356
Seventh	Pumpkin seeds	1 ounce	333

SOURCE: USDA National Nutrient Database for Standard Reference, Release 24

Honorable mentions: Parmesan cheese, beef, eggs, chicken, mozzarella

Best food groups: Meat, seafood, dairy, nuts and seeds, whole-grain products

What is phosphorus and why is it so important? Phosphorus is the second-most-abundant mineral in the body, next to calcium. It works in concert with calcium and other minerals to form bone and support cell structure. Most of phosphorus (about 85 percent) is located in bones; the rest is helping the body filter out waste, storing and using energy, and producing the genetic material, DNA.

Documented cases of phosphorus deficiencies (hypophosphatemia) are usually quite rare because of its abundance in the food supply, unless intake is low due to starvation. Hypophosphatemia is also seen in health conditions that cause phosphorus to be poorly absorbed or wasted, such as alcoholism, diabetes, and anorexia nervosa. Deficiency symptoms include loss of appetite, anemia, muscle weakness, bone pain, rickets (in children), osteomalacia (in adults), increased susceptibility to infection, numbness and tingling of the extremities, fatigue, and even death.

Did you know? Matches, tracer bullets, and fireworks are all made from red phosphorus! Other popular uses of phosphorus are to make fertilizer; glassware; and trisodium phosphate, which is used as a cleaner, water softener, and corrosion inhibitor. Calcium phosphate, also known as bone ash, is used to make chinaware and baking powder.

HOW MUCH IS ENOUGH?

The DV for phosphorus is 1,000 mg, based on a 2,000-calorie diet.

Dietary Reference Intakes (DRIs) for Phosphorus

Age	Children (mg/day)	Males (mg/day)	Females (mg/day)	Pregnancy (mg/day)	Lactation (mg/day)
0–6 months	100				
6–12 months	275				
1–3 years	460				
4–8 years	500				
9–13 years		1,250	1,250		
14–18 years		1,250	1,250	1,250	1,250
19–50 years		700	700	700	700
51+ years		700	700		

SOURCE: Food and Nutrition Board, Institutes of Medicine, National Academies

Too much! The UL for adults is 4,000 mg per day and toxicity is not generally seen in healthy people consuming 3,000 mg per day. Elevated phosphorus levels can be seen in unstable hospitalized patients and those with poor kidney function. Aside from being identified on a blood test, there are no symptoms. High phosphate levels can effect bone mineralization and negatively affect blood calcium levels.

Supplement it? Not necessary—plenty of foods to meet one's needs.

First Place: Ricotta Cheese

Technically, ricotta is not even cheese! It is almost entirely made up of whey, a by-product of the cheese-making process. In Italian, *ricotta* means "re-cooked"; the whey is originally in liquid form and must be cooked down to make it into ricotta cheese. Nonfat ricotta is also an excellent source of calcium and a good source of vitamin A. Because of its origins in whey, ricotta has a higher biological-value protein than cottage cheese, which is mostly made up from the protein casein. Whey also has higher branch chain amino acid content, which is beneficial for stimulating lean muscle growth.

Shocker Food! ———————————————————————

Soda is a shocker because it's *not* a significant source of phosphorus as it is often touted to be! For example, one 12-ounce can of a popular cola beverage contains only 69 mg of this mineral; you would need to chug down about three cans for the drink to even be considered an excellent source. Bottom line: Don't look to soda to meet any of your nutritional needs!

First Runner-Up: Soybeans

Get the scoop on this nutrient-rich legume on page 291. Although whole soy has the highest level of phosphorus, the content in soy milk is greatly reduced—about half the amount of phosphorus than you would find in cow's milk.

Second Runner-Up: Sardines

Read more about this healthy fish on page 291. Sardines are the perfect food for building bones because of their triple threat of calcium, phosphorus, and vitamin D!

Fourth: Beef Liver

Learn more about this healthy organ meat on page 286. The bioavailability (ability to be absorbed) of phosphorus differs, depending on the food source. Research shows that phosphorus absorption is higher from meat sources than from plant sources. Meat in general is high in phosphorus, but other commonly consumed livers did not come close to beef liver.

Fifth: Lentils

For more about the benefits of this tiny legume, see page 289. Do not eat undercooked (crunchy) lentils; they contain phytic acid, which makes it hard for your body to absorb phosphorus. Undercooked lentils may cause gastric distress, too.

Sixth: Yogurt

A study in Japan found that those adolescents who consumed more phosphorus-rich dairy products, such as yogurt, had the highest bone density, compared to those who didn't consume many dairy products at all. Go with low-fat plain yogurt, for the most nutrition (see page 292) minus the sugar and cholesterol of other varieties.

Seventh: Pumpkin Seeds

Pumpkin seeds are an excellent source of copper, manganese, magnesium, and phosphorus, and a good source of iron and zinc. Animal research suggests that consuming pumpkin seeds regularly helps reduce benign prostatic hyperplasia, otherwise known as a swollen prostate gland. Because of their high phosphorus content, eating pumpkin seeds may help reduce the incidence of bladder stones.

TOP 7 SOURCES OF POTASSIUM

SNEAK-A-PEEK: RANKINGS AT A GLANCE

Ranking	Food	Serving	Amount (mg)
First Place	**Beet greens (cooked)**	**1 cup**	**1,310**
First Runner-Up	**White beans (cooked)**	**1 cup**	**1,190**
Second Runner-Up	**Soybeans (cooked)**	**1 cup**	**970**
Fourth	Lima beans (cooked)	1 cup	955
Fifth	Spinach (cooked)	1 cup	839
Sixth	Sweet potatoes (cooked)	1 cup	796
Seventh	Lentils (cooked)	1 cup	731

SOURCE: USDA National Nutrient Database for Standard Reference, Release 24

Honorable mentions: Tomato paste, puree, and sauce; bananas and plantains; tropical trail mix; halibut; tuna; cod; chocolate milk

Best food groups: Vegetables, dairy, fish, fruits

What is potassium and why is it so important? Without it, our heart would cease to beat! Potassium is one of the most important minerals, as it is required by every cell to function properly. Potassium helps keep our body's pH levels perfectly balanced—not too acidic, not too alkaline. Deficiencies in potassium have also been attributed to heart arrhythmias, muscle cramps and weakness, high blood pressure, glucose intolerance, kidney stones, bone loss, cardiovascular disease, stroke, and death.

Did you know? Some SAD (standard American diet) facts: The average American adult consumes only 2,750 mg of potassium daily—about 58 percent of what is considered an adequate intake. So, if you are like most, you may need up to an additional 2,000 mg of potassium every day. Of course, this will vary, depending on your intake and unique needs. Those who are on prescription drugs, such as potassium-wasting diuretics for controlling fluid balance and blood pressure, or who are experiencing diarrhea or vomiting, or who sweat excessively, may require higher levels.

HOW MUCH IS ENOUGH?

The DV for potassium is 3,500 mg, based on a 2,000-calorie diet.

Dietary Reference Intakes (DRIs) for Potassium

Age	Children (mg/day)	Males (mg/day)	Females (mg/day)	Pregnancy (mg/day)	Lactation (mg/day)
0–6 months	400				
6–12 months	700				
1–3 years	3,000				
4–8 years	3,800				
9–13 years		4,500	4,500		
14–18 years		4,700	4,700	4,700	5,100
19–50 years		4,700	4,700	4,700	5,100
51+ years		4,700	4,700		

SOURCE: Food and Nutrition Board, Institutes of Medicine, National Academies

Too much! Consuming very high levels of potassium has been linked to heart attacks! To date, no UL for potassium has been established, and rarely has excessive potassium been achieved through dietary intake alone.

Supplement it? Potassium can be found in multivitamins, individual supplements, and sports beverages. The highest dose available is 99 mg. Ingesting too much potassium can be life threatening, so you should always consult your doctor or registered dietitian before taking supplements containing potassium.

First Place: Beet Greens

Beet greens are an excellent source of potassium. See page 288 for the other goodies offered by these deep green sprouts.

> Ten to 15 percent of the population may have a red or pink tinge in their urine after eating beet greens. This harmless condition is known as beeturia, whereby some people may not be able to break down the flavonoid betacyanin, the pigment that causes the color change. The same effect may be had by eating the beets themselves.

First Runner-Up: White Beans

Whether purchased dried and cooked or ready-to-eat in the can, white beans contain the same nutrition value (see page 286). White beans are an excellent source of potassium.

Shocker Food!

Did you know that French fries also provide a good source of potassium (731 mg in a medium-size serving)? Yes—fries have as much potassium as lentils, and believe it or not, more than a medium-size baked potato! And yes, traditional fries also bring along extra fat and sodium, but that can be controlled: Quick-frozen fries can be baked to avoid extra oil, and just a bit of salt can do the trick. Bottom line—French not-fried fries can be a healthy choice for getting potassium into the diet. PS: If you make them yourself, eat the skin! You will find lots of potassium and 50 percent of the vitamin C located in the skin of the potato. Total shocker!

Second Runner-Up: Soybeans

Yes, here it is again, the wonder bean (see page 291). Soybeans are nearly the top of the list when it comes to supplying potassium.

Fourth: Lima Beans

Besides being an excellent source of heart-healthy potassium and fiber (see page 286 for even more goodies offered by this legume), lima beans may also offer anticancer properties, as they are rich in the phytochemicals coumestrol and saponin.

Fifth: Spinach

Spinach is probably one of the best vegetables on earth for the heart. Besides all of its vitamins and minerals like potassium (see page 291 for the lineup), the flavonoids and nitrates in spinach help lower blood pressure and keeps blood flowing through arteries that feed the heart and every other part of the body. A randomized study supports that subjects who ate spinach had improved endothelial function: lower blood pressure.

Sixth: Sweet Potato

Besides potassium and a host of other vitamins and minerals (see page 291), sweet potatoes, especially the purple varieties, are also rich in carotenoids and anthocyanins. This combination of plant nutrients plus potassium helps assist in lowering blood pressure and improve heart health.

Seventh: Lentils

Lentils' high fiber and nutrient composition, including potassium (see page 289 for a fuller list), makes it an optimal legume for combating heart disease. A study that included a calorie-controlled diet that served legumes, such as lentils, four times per week for eight weeks, showed a reduction in inflammatory markers such as C-reactive protein, as well as significant improvement in lipids and blood pressure in overweight and obese subjects.

TOP 7 SOURCES OF SELENIUM

SNEAK-A-PEEK: RANKINGS AT A GLANCE

Ranking	Food	Serving	Amount (mcg)
First Place	**Brazil nuts**	**1 ounce**	**543**
First Runner-Up	**Yellowfin tuna (cooked)**	**3 ounces**	**92**
Second Runner-Up	**Orange roughy (cooked)**	**3 ounces**	**75**
Fourth	Rockfish (cooked)	3 ounces	64.8
Fifth	Lobster (cooked)	3 ounces	62
Sixth	Swordfish (cooked)	3 ounces	58
Seventh	Oysters (cooked)	3 ounces	56

SOURCE: USDA National Nutrient Database for Standard Reference, Release 24

Honorable mentions: Herring, flounder, perch, halibut, clams, turkey, yeast

Best food groups: Fish, nuts

What is selenium and why is it so important? Selenium is a trace mineral (meaning your body only needs small amounts) that has powerful antioxidant properties and may play a role in fighting cancer. It assists in producing antioxidant proteins that protect cells from free radical damage. Aside from being a great antioxidant, selenium also boosts immune function. Observational studies have found that those who include foods higher in selenium have lower rates of lung, colorectal, and prostate cancers. A French study of over two hundred elderly men and women found those who consumed more selenium-rich foods, such as seafood, had measureable health benefits, such as better brain health and improved blood profiles. Women and men who are HIV-positive often present with a selenium deficiency, which is thought to speed up the progression of the disease. Research has shown that eating high-selenium foods or taking selenium supplements may help slow down the progression of HIV and increase chances of survival.

Selenium deficiency is rarely seen in the United States; however, there are serious conditions where deficiencies do occur: Kashin-Beck disease (which results in osteoarthropathy), Keshan disease (most often seen in selenium-deficient children), enlarged heart and compromised heart function, and myxedematous endemic cretinism (results in mental retardation).

Did you know? The highest concentrations of selenium in the body are located in the thyroid, kidneys, muscles, and liver.

HOW MUCH IS ENOUGH?

The DV for selenium is 70 mcg, based on a 2,000-calorie diet.

Dietary Reference Intakes (DRIs) for Selenium

Age	Children (mg/day)	Males (mg/day)	Females (mg/day)	Pregnancy (mg/day)	Lactation (mg/day)
0–6 months	15				
6–12 months	20				
1–3 years	20				
4–8 years	30				
9–13 years		40	40		
14–18 years		55	55	60	70
19–50 years		55	55	60	70
51+ years		55	55		

SOURCE: Food and Nutrition Board, Institutes of Medicine, National Academies

Too much! Toxic levels of selenium can sometimes give off a garlic smell that can be detected on the breath. Selenium toxicity has been associated with dermatitis, loose hair, and diseased nails, and some studies suggest that high levels of selenium in the diet can be a risk factor for type 2 diabetes. The National Academy of Sciences has set a UL for selenium at 400 mg per day for adults.

Supplement it? Selenium in the form of selenomethionine is absorbed 100 percent. Other forms of selenium supplements are not as efficiently absorbed. Selenium supplements come in capsules and tablets and are usually a component of multivitamins.

First Place: Brazil Nuts

A 1-ounce serving of this nut has over 750 percent of our selenium daily needs! The rest of the top seven foods don't even come close! The selenium in Brazil nuts positively impacts male testosterone levels and boosts sperm movement and production. Brazil nuts are also the highest in saturated fat out of all other nuts. Turn to page 286 to learn more about this incredible nut.

> The Brazil nut tree is among the highest trees in the rainforest, reaching heights of 165 feet tall, and can live for as long as a thousand years.

First Runner-Up: Yellowfin Tuna

Along with being nutrient-rich in a variety of other ways (see page 292), yellowfin tuna, canned in water, is an excellent source of selenium. Selenium protects the body from mercury, cadmium, and silver poisoning. This is helpful especially in those fish found with higher levels of mercury, such as tuna.

Second Runner-Up: Orange Roughy

> The orange roughy was originally named "slimehead." I can't imagine how sales were before the name change!

Several marine societies have placed the orange roughy on their "do not eat" list because the species is becoming endangered worldwide. Besides being high in selenium, it is low in fat and an excellent source of protein.

Fourth: Rockfish

The term *rockfish* can refer to a number of fish, but a more familiar name is striped bass. Whatever you call it, rockfish is an excellent source of selenium and other nutrients (see page 290).

Fifth: Lobster

Lobster is an excellent source of selenium. Learn more about lobster on page 289.

Sixth: Swordfish

While every fish has some level of mercury, swordfish, along with shark, king mackerel, tuna, and other large predatory fish, contain high amounts of mercury. This is

After lobsters molt and lose their shell, they are so hungry that they often eat the shell they just came from! By doing this, their calcium is replenished, which helps harden their new shell.

why the Environmental Defense Fund recommends that women and children under age twelve should not eat swordfish, and men should only eat it once a month, due to such high levels of mercury. That said, swordfish is an excellent source of selenium and other nutrients (see page 291). A study of over eight thousand adults found that those who included ample anti-oxidant foods such as swordfish had lower levels of the inflammatory markers C-reactive protein and homocysteine.

Swordfish have been reported to be up to 15 feet long and weighing up to 1,400 pounds! Out of twenty-five thousand fish species, only twenty-two of these cold-blooded animals have the ability to "heat their eyes"—including swordfish.

Seventh: Oysters

Selenium-rich foods, such as oysters, help produce in the body a powerful antioxidant called glutathione, which is known to help protect against certain types of cancer. Turn to page 289 for more about oysters' benefits.

TOP 7 SOURCES OF SODIUM

SNEAK-A-PEEK: RANKINGS AT A GLANCE

Ranking	Food	Serving	Amount (mg)
First Place	Crab (cooked)	3 ounces	914
First Runner-Up	Table salt	¼ teaspoon	581
Second Runner-Up	Clams (raw)	3 ounces	511
Fourth	Lobster (cooked)	3 ounces	413
Fifth	Walleye (cooked)	3 ounces	356
Sixth	Beet greens (cooked)	1 cup	347
Seventh	Cod (cooked)	3 ounces	316

SOURCE: USDA National Nutrient Database for Standard Reference, Release 24

Honorable mentions: Swiss chard, canned foods, processed meats, frozen entrées and side dishes, cheese, snacks and other processed foods

Best food groups: Salt, greens

What is sodium and why is it so important? First, let's set the record straight. Sodium is not a *bad* thing. How could it be, when it's required by every single cell of every animal on earth! Some may argue about its over-abundance in the Western diet, but sodium shouldn't be targeted for annihilation; rather, moderation! Along with the mineral potassium, sodium is responsible for stimulating and carrying electrical impulses along nerve and muscle tissue. It also plays a large role in the kidney by maintaining fluid balance in the body.

When sodium levels dip too low, a condition referred to as hyponatremia occurs, causing the cells in the body to swell, which can lead to mild to severe health problems, even death.

Did you know? The most common form of sodium in our diet is called sodium chloride, a.k.a. salt, which contains about 40 percent sodium. Sodium chloride has many uses, including preserving and drying out foods. It is estimated that the average American man consumes upward of 4,700 mg of sodium per day; and the average woman upward of 3,100 mg, assuming a lower calorie intake for women compared to men. Ironically, the salt shaker is not the major contributor of sodium in the diet—it is sodium chloride that has been added to processed foods. While it may be true that too much salt can lead to potential health problems, those who have low blood pressure (hypotension) may benefit by adding salt to their diet.

HOW MUCH IS ENOUGH?

The DV for sodium is 2,400 mg, based on a 2,000-calorie diet.

Dietary Reference Intakes (DRIs) for Sodium

Age	Children (g/day)	Males (g/day)	Females (g/day)	Pregnancy (g/day)	Lactation (g/day)
0–6 months	0.12				
7–12 months	0.37				
1–3 years	1.0				
4–8 years	1.2				
9–13 years		1.5	1.5		
14–18 years		1.5	1.5	1.5	1.5
19–50 years		1.5	1.5	1.5	1.5
55+ years		1.5	1.5		

SOURCE: Food and Nutrition Board, Institutes of Medicine, National Academies

Too much! The prevailing yet still controversial wisdom is that people should not consume more than 2,300 mg per day, the equivalent of about 1 teaspoon of salt. According to the CDC, "Reducing sodium intake to 2,300 mg per day potentially could prevent 11 million cases of hypertension and save billions of dollars in health-care expenditures; reducing sodium intake further would yield additional benefits." However, those who fall into certain categories based on age, ethnicity, or health challenge may benefit from capping their intake at 1,500 mg. These groups include anyone over the age of fifty; African Americans; and those afflicted with high blood pressure, metabolic syndrome, heart disease, and kidney disease. The average person in the United States consumes more than enough sodium, based on these recommendations, than is necessary due to our yearning for processed food. As a safeguard mechanism, the kidneys can normally control the amount of sodium in the blood; however, if a person consumes too much sodium over time, it can take its toll on blood pressure, bone health, and even kidney health. Just like the effects of sodium deficiency, if more sodium is consumed than the kidneys can handle, fluid retention will result. Eventually, this process will lead to high blood pressure causing a myriad of health complications including heart and kidney failure and other vascular diseases.

Supplement it? Sodium pills can be purchased over-the-counter at pharmacies, but this should only be used if you have hypotension or are an athlete who is prone to "salty sweater syndrome," which is excessive sodium loss through perspiration. Seek professional guidance in either scenario.

Shocker Food!

A dinner of six to eight medium-size breaded and fried shrimp contains 1,875 mg of sodium—that's without fries or cocktail sauce!

First Place: Crab

Crab is naturally salty because it lives in seawater. See page 104 for other nutritional information about sodium. In a randomized study, twenty-three healthy men were given 225 grams of crab or shrimp to eat every day for twelve weeks. Cholesterol was drawn before and after the test. Neither of the diets raised total or LDL cholesterol.

First Runner-Up: Table Salt

Most table salt is fortified with iodine to ensure that individuals receive enough in their diet to avoid goiters and avert hypothyroidism; however, there is a growing trend toward using sea salt and other designer salts that are not always fortified with iodine. One-quarter teaspoon of salt provides 71 mg of iodine. See all about iodine on page 72.

> About 40 percent of global use of salt is by industry for the purpose of making chlorine and soda ash. Other uses for sodium chloride include water softening and roadside salt to make icy roads safe.

Second Runner-Up: Clams

Clams are not only rich in sodium but numerous other nutrients (see page 287). Two animal studies found that when rats that had elevated cholesterol were fed a diet enhanced with extract from fresh clams, their cholesterol reduced significantly and so did incidence of fatty liver. Human research is need for this promising extract.

Fourth: Lobster

Yet another seafood, lobster is rich in sodium, as well as other vitamins and minerals (see page 289).

> Ever wonder if something could be done with left over lobster shells? The shells of crustaceans are rich in a substance called chitosan, which has been used commercially to sop up oil spills and also on the home front as a dietary fat absorber. However, chitosan's effectiveness for weight loss is questionable. There's also lots of calcium in lobster shells: Japanese researchers were able to reverse osteoporosis in lab rats by adding powdered lobster shell to their diet for six weeks.

Fifth: Walleye

Walleye is a fresh-water fish native to North America and is an excellent source of phosphorus, protein, selenium, and vitamin B$_{12}$, and a good source of choline, niacin, and potassium. The Wisconsin Department of Natural Resources found that mercury levels rose nearly 19 percent in walleye between 1982 and 2005 and recommends that women of childbearing age and children younger than age fifteen should limit their walleye intake to no more than one serving a month. One study, measuring fish consumption, found that as walleye consumption increased, the serum levels of PCBs also increased. Walleye might not want to eat that! Sorry . . . couldn't resist.

Sixth: Beet Greens

How can something that grows from the ground be high in sodium? Both beet greens and Swiss chard belong to the same plant family but for some unknown reason, beet greens are much higher in sodium! However, ironically, a British study found that those who drank 500 ml of beet juice had a significant lowering of blood pressure hours later, possibly due to the nitric oxide content of beets. The authors of the study said the results were as effective as if the subjects received oral nitrate supplements. See page 288 for the other benefits of beet greens.

Seventh: Cod

Aside from cod being a great source of sodium, a Norwegian study found that children who ate cod, as opposed to taking cod liver oil, had fewer cases of eczema. It was determined that eating cod early in life was more important than Mom's maternal consumption of cod in an effort to prevent eczema in her children.

TOP 7 SOURCES OF ZINC

SNEAK-A-PEEK: RANKINGS AT A GLANCE

Ranking	Food	Serving Size	Amount (mg)
First Place	Oysters (fried) (raw)	3 ounces 3 ounces	74 33
First Runner-Up	Beef (cooked)	3 ounces	8.73
Second Runner-Up	Alaskan king crab (cooked)	3 ounces	6.5

continues

continued

Ranking	Food	Serving Size	Amount (mg)
Fourth	Lamb (cooked)	3 ounces	6.2
Fifth	Pork (cooked)	3 ounces	3.91
Sixth	Turkey (cooked)	3 ounces	3.75
Seventh	Lobster (cooked)	3 ounces	3.44

SOURCE: USDA National Nutrient Database for Standard Reference, Release 24

Honorable mentions: Baked beans, ricotta cheese, wheat germ, fortified cereal

Best food groups: Meat, shellfish

What is zinc and why is it so important? The importance of zinc for human health was first identified and written about in 1963. Zinc is all about wound healing and bolstering your defenses—especially the immune system—and is an essential mineral in all stages of procreation, as well as promoting normal growth throughout the life cycle. It helps fight off troublesome bacteria and viruses while supporting and protecting DNA, the genetic computer code of your body. Zinc also contributes to your sense of taste and smell. Deficiencies in zinc may bring about growth retardation, loss of appetite, impaired immune function, hair loss, diarrhea, delayed sexual maturation, impotence and infertility, hypogonadism in males, eye and skin lesions, weight loss, delayed healing of wounds, taste abnormalities, and lethargy.

Did you know? Adequate zinc can be found in a balanced diet; however, for many Americans, balanced is a challenging concept, especially when it comes to diet and lifestyle behaviors. Vegetarians or those with digestive malabsorption may have a higher risk of developing a zinc deficiency.

Shocker Food!

Contrary to the popular belief that swallowing watermelon seeds whole will cause a melon to grow in your stomach, what they will do, if you chew them up, is provide such nutrients as iron, magnesium, phosphorus, protein, and zinc. A 1-ounce serving contains 3 mg of zinc.

HOW MUCH IS ENOUGH?

The DV for zinc is 15 mg, based on a 2,000-calorie diet.

Dietary Reference Intakes (DRIs) of Zinc

Age	Children (mg/day)	Males (mg/day)	Females (mg/day)	Pregnancy (mg/day)	Lactation (mg/day)
0–6 months	2				
7–12 months	3				
1–3 years	3				
4–8 years	5				
9–13 years		8	8		
14–18 years		11	9	12	13
19+ years		11	8	11	12

SOURCE: Food and Nutrition Board, Institutes of Medicine, National Academies

Too much! The UL has been set at 40 mg per day for all adults. Although rare in a healthy population, toxicity cases have been reported. Short-term symptoms include nausea or vomiting, low appetite, diarrhea, and headache. Long-term symptoms include copper deficiency and reduced immune function.

Supplement it? The most common form of zinc supplementation is as a tablet or capsule. Most multivitamins contain zinc. You can also find zinc in lozenge or syrup form, which may be particularly beneficial for reducing the duration and severity of the common cold if taken within 24 hours of onset of symptoms. A recent review of seventeen studies found that those who took zinc supplements knocked an average of three days off their cold!

First Place: Oysters

Read more about these mollusks on page 289. Including zinc-rich foods such as oysters in a healthy diet may play a role in fighting chronic diseases such as cancer, diabetes, depression, Wilson's disease, Alzheimer's disease, and other age-related diseases.

> Oysters can live to be one hundred years old,
> but most that we consume are mere youngsters,
> between three and five years, when the meat is
> at its best quality.

First Runner-Up: Beef

See page 286 for the healthy benefits of beef. The common misconception may be that this meat is loaded with fat. However, lean roast beef has less than 5 g of fat per 3-ounce serving. It was found in a study that the consumption of lean beef contributed significantly to the intake of zinc and other key nutrients without increasing intakes of total fat, saturated fatty acids, or sodium.

Second Runner-Up: Alaskan King Crab

Turn to page 287 for more about this tasty crustacean. Don't be fooled by *imitation* crab, though, which has less of these nutrients and is made mostly of artificially flavored pollack! A study found

> The world is full of crabs! Can you believe there are over four thousand varieties? The most popular in the United States are the blue (mainly on the East Coast) and Dungeness (mainly on the West Coast) varieties.

that poor zinc status could contribute to insulin resistance in children. Eating zinc-rich foods, such as crab, as part of a good diet could improve the health and nutritional status of children and reduce the risk for diabetes.

Fourth: Lamb

To see the many benefits of lamb, see page 289. The average American consumes less than a pound of lamb a year—usually just for holiday dinners! Eating more lamb than the average American may make you happier, as low dietary intake of zinc was more strongly associated with depression!

(As with other animal protein, there are healthy and less healthy cuts, so choose leaner varieties.)

Fifth: Pork

Turn to page 290 for more about pork. A Danish study found that young women who consumed a diet that included lean pork had higher blood zinc levels than did those who ate a vegetarian diet. Zinc is more bioavailable from animal products than it is from plant sources.

Sixth: Turkey

Turkey, in general, is a good source of iron, riboflavin, thiamine, and vitamins B_6 and B_{12}, but the dark meat has a slightly higher concentration of these micronutrients and a bit more fat. Three ounces of cooked skinless light and dark meat has about 2 and 5 g of fat, respectively. Studies have suggested that by eating zinc-rich foods such as turkey, pregnant women may lower their child's risk of childhood asthma.

> About 90 percent of Americans eat turkey on Thanksgiving, and according to the U.S. Census Bureau, over 248 million turkeys were raised in 2011.

Seventh: Lobster

Besides containing zinc, lobster is also an excellent source of other nutrients (see page 289). The high phytate content of grains are known to decrease the bioavailability of zinc. Make sure you include in your diet high-biological-value zinc sources, such as lobster and other animal proteins, or take a zinc supplement to assure adequate zinc status.

CHAPTER 3
Chewing the Fats, Fiber, and Phytosterols

TOP 7 SOURCES OF MONOUNSATURATED FATS

SNEAK-A-PEEK: RANKINGS AT A GLANCE

Ranking	Food	Serving	Amount (g)
First Place	Macadamia nuts (roasted)	1 ounce	17.0
First Runner-Up	Hazelnuts	1 ounce	13.0
Second Runner-Up	Pecans	1 ounce	11.6
Fourth	Safflower oil	1 tablespoon	10.2
Fifth	Herring (cooked or pickled)	3 ounces	10.16
Sixth	Olive oil	1 tablespoon	9.9
Seventh	Canola oil	1 tablespoon	8.9

SOURCE: USDA National Nutrient Database for Standard Reference, Release 24

Honorable mentions: Soybean oil, almonds, peanuts, cashews, avocados

Best food groups? Nuts, oils, fish

What are monounsaturated fats and why are they so important? They are called monounsaturated because their chemical structure includes one (mono) double-bonded (unsaturated) carbon molecule. This fat is also

113

known as MUFA, short for monounsaturated fatty acid. Two different types of monounsaturated fats are found in the diet: palmitoleic and oleic acid. Palmitoleic acid is what you would find in macadamia nuts and animal fats. Although those aren't foods we often think about as being healthy, research has demonstrated that people with higher levels of palmitoleic acid had healthier levels of blood cholesterol, inflammatory markers, insulin levels, and insulin sensitivity. Even though there isn't a heart-health claim allowed for macadamia nuts, diets that included 1.5 ounces a day were as effective in reducing cholesterol as was a standard heart-healthy diet. Oleic acid is what is found in plant foods, such as olive oil and nuts.

Did you know? Monounsaturated fats are the only type of fats known to lower LDL and total cholesterol while, at the same time, thought to raise protective HDL cholesterol (see page 162).

How much is enough? Eighteen to 28 percent of your total fats should be made up of monounsaturated and polyunsaturated fats. Based on a 2,000-calorie diet, that translates into no more that 16 g of saturated fats, less than 2 g of trans fats, and somewhere between 50 and 70 g of monos and polys combined.

Too much! Extra fat, even the good stuff, just spells extra calories . . . which often lead to weight gain! Most health experts recommend you not exceed 35 percent of your calories from total fat.

Shocker Food!

Pork, lamb, and beef ribs range from 10.26 to 11.46 g of monos per 3-ounce cooked portion. Although they technically deserve a place in the top 7, they are also high in saturated fat and cholesterol; therefore, the nasty fats outweigh the healthy attributes of their monounsaturated fat content. Whole-milk ricotta cheese should have ranked in the top 7 as well, but again it's debatable whether it should be allowed, because of the saturated fat company it keeps. I suggest sticking with mainly lean cuts of meat and low-fat dairy products and getting most of your MUFAs from the top 7.

Supplement it? Food sources of MUFAs are both plentiful and delicious, so supplementation isn't necessary.

First Place: Macadamia Nuts

Dry-roasted macadamia nuts deliver the highest source of monounsaturated fats of any known food. Roasting them increases their nutrient density because water is removed in the process. They are also an excellent source of manganese and a good source of thiamine and fiber. And you'll find heart-healthy phytosterols in macadamia nuts, which play an important role in reducing cholesterol levels and promoting prostate health. Macadamia nuts contain high amounts of the amino acid arginine, which helps promote nitric oxide, expanding arteries to allow for easy blood flow. Less restricted blood flow means less chance for blood clots and stroke. A small, randomized study showed better reduction in total and LDL cholesterol in the macadamia-munching group compared to the control group that skipped the nuts.

First Runner-Up: Hazelnuts

Turn to page 288 for the fuller story about hazelnuts, which are an excellent source of monounsaturated fat. Eat them whole and raw! A study found that many of the health-beneficial nutrients of this nut are contained within the skin instead of the flesh. Roasting was found to diminish the nutrition content slightly.

> The hazelnut is the official state nut of Oregon. Over 95 percent of the U.S. production of this nut occurs in Oregon's Willamette Valley.

Second Runner-Up: Pecans

Pecans are a good source of fiber and contain more than nineteen vitamins and minerals, as well as monounsaturated fat. They also contain heart disease–fighting phytosterols. Diets high in nuts, including pecans, have been shown to reduce C-reactive protein and inflammatory marker that has been associated with an increased risk for stroke, heart attacks, and circulatory diseases. A 2011 study that appeared in the *Journal of Nutrition* showed that a pecan-enriched diet was nearly twice as effective in dropping total and bad (LDL) cholesterol, compared to the low-fat Step 1 diet.

Fourth: Safflower Oil

Safflower oil, also an excellent source of vitamin E, is a great healthy substitute for other vegetable oils or butter because it is high in monounsaturated fat, while extremely low in saturated fat and no cholesterol. Additionally, it is flavorless and colorless, so it's perfect when trying to maintain the flavor of a dish. If you need to deep-fry, high-oleic safflower oil is one of the best oils, because it retains nutrients to a high smoke point of 509°F. An Ohio State University study found that a daily 8 g (about 1.5 teaspoons) serving of safflower oil improved blood glucose control, inflammation, and blood lipids in fifty-five diabetic women over the course of sixteen weeks.

Fifth: Herring

Herring are actually grown-up sardines! They are a fatty fish, just like salmon, tuna, and mackerel. Herring is actually twice as high in EPA (a heart-healthy omega-3) than salmon; however, salmon is four times higher in DHA (the other heart-healthy omega-3) than herring. It is also an excellent source of niacin, phosphorus, riboflavin, selenium, and vitamins B_6 and B_{12}, not to mention being a good source of eight other vitamins and minerals. The University of Maryland Medical Center points to the Inuit for the health benefits of fatty fish, highlighting their low incidence of colon cancer. UMMC also revealed that these omega-3 rich fish can help reduce or slow the progression of other cancers, including breast and prostate.

Sixth: Olive Oil

A staple ingredient in the Mediterranean diet, extra-virgin olive oil is the real stuff you want. Unlike most vegetable oils, olive oil should be consumed in its crude, unprocessed form. This means no heat treatment or machine harvesting, otherwise the delicate compounds that give olive oil that heart health seal of approval are destroyed and/or removed. Olive oil is also good source of vitamin E and contains maslinic and oleanolic acids, which researchers have shown prevent human colon cancer cells from multiplying and restore cellular function. Substituting this liquid gold for an equivalent amount of other fats or oils can help reduce an individual's risk for heart disease.

Seventh: Canola Oil

Canola oil, though often mistaken for its cousin rapeseed oil (not to be confused with grapeseed oil; see page 120), does not contain the strong-tasting glucosinolates and potentially harmful erucic acid like rapeseed oil does. Canola also contains the lowest level of saturated fats of any vegetable oil and is an excellent source of monounsaturated and omega-3 fatty acids, which produce healthy cholesterol levels. Like corn oil, canola is also a rich source of vitamin E. In a small three-week, randomized study, subjects with elevated cholesterol were placed on two different diets: one that contained dairy fat, and another that replaced dairy fat with canola oil. The canola oil diet reduced the levels of serum cholesterol by 17 percent, triglycerides by 20 percent, and LDL cholesterol by 17 percent.

TOP 7 SOURCES OF POLYUNSATURATED FATS

SNEAK-A-PEEK: RANKINGS AT A GLANCE

Ranking	Food	Serving	Amount (mg)
First Place	Walnuts	1 ounce	13.4
	Walnut oil	1 tablespoon	8.6
First Runner-Up	Pine nuts	1 ounce	9.7
Second Runner-Up	Grapeseed oil	1 tablespoon	9.5
Fourth	Sunflower seeds	1 ounce	9.2
	Sunflower oil	1 tablespoon	8.9
Fifth	Flaxseed oil	1 tablespoon	9.2
Sixth	Soybeans	1 cup	8.7
Seventh	Corn oil	1 tablespoon	7.4

SOURCE: USDA National Nutrient Database for Standard Reference, Release 24

Honorable mentions: Pecans, Brazil nuts, sesame oil, pumpkin seeds

Best food groups: Nuts and seeds, and their oils

What is polyunsaturated fat and why is it so important? Polyunsaturated fatty acids, or PUFA for short, contain at least two double bonds (poly) on its fatty-acid carbon chain. PUFAs are essential fatty acids (meaning our body can't make them), and include omega-3 fatty acids (EPA, DHA, ALA) and omega-6 fatty acids (linoleic acid). You'd probably know one if you saw one, as polyunsaturated fats are typically liquid at room temperature and even when they are refrigerated. One function of these in the body is to produce another type of fatty acid called arachidonic acid, which controls the signaling pathways that are responsible for regulating the body's warning system; namely, the inflammation response.

Did you know? PUFAs have been shown to reduce cholesterol levels, and in turn lower the risk for heart disease, when substituted for saturated fats.

How much is enough? As noted earlier, it is recommended to consume 25 to 35 percent of your calories from fat: no more than 10 percent of fat from saturated fat, with the rest split up evenly between polyunsaturated and monounsaturated fat. Polyunsaturated fats are pretty prevalent in the diet, so it is nearly impossible for someone of average health and appetite to be deficient in PUFAs. However, most health experts agree there is way too much omega-6 fatty acids and not enough omega-3s in the American diet.

Too much! A lot of literature on inflammation details the perils of overconsumption of omega-6s. These "diseases of civilization," which include type 2 diabetes, stroke, Alzheimer's disease, heart disease, and many others, have links to suboptimal distribution of healthy fats in our diet. That is, the high levels of omega-6s wouldn't be a problem if we consumed adequate levels of omega-3s to balance them out.

Supplement it? Polyunsaturated fats are plentiful in the diet, but as mentioned earlier, most people would benefit from increasing their omega-3. See page 121 for more guidance.

Shocker Food!

The number one highest source of polyunsaturated fat listed in the USDA reference 24 database is piecrust, due to its high fat content. It's great to know that Grandma's traditional lard crust has been replaced by healthier fats, but unless you have been living under a rock and didn't get the memo, piecrust is *not* considered a healthy food.

First Place: Walnuts and Walnut Oil

Walnuts are the richest source of omega-3s compared to any other nut, an excellent source of copper and manganese, and a good source of iron, magnesium, and phosphorus. Don't remove that skin. The skin contains about 90 percent of the nuts' phenols, which include phenolic acids, flavonoids, and tannins. Walnuts are also an excellent source of vitamin E, particularly a form called gamma-tocopherol, which a study showed may reduce the growth of colon cancer cells in vitro. Researchers from Penn State found that by adding a combination of walnut oil and walnuts to the diet reduced resting diastolic blood pressure even during times of stress.

The walnut is the oldest nut known to mankind, dating back to 7000 BC. English walnuts, which are the most commonly consumed walnut in America, were originally reserved only for the royal family in ancient Persia. English merchants transported the nuts for trade around the world, where they were referred to as "English walnuts," though they were never grown commercially in England. California produces most of the world's supply of walnuts.

First Runner-Up: Pine Nuts

Pine nuts are an excellent source of PUFAs, as well as other nutrients . . . if you're not allergic to them (see page 88). Moreover, the oil in pine nuts might be the best thing since paper napkins for controlling hunger: Researchers found that Korean pine nut oil stimulates two appetite-suppressant hormones called cholecystokinin and GLP-1. Women subjects who ingested the oil reported significantly suppressed appetite thirty minutes after ingestion!

Second Runner-Up: Grapeseed Oil

Grapeseed oil has a smoke point of 420°F, making it an ideal cooking oil. Its high polyunsaturated content and clean, light taste allows it to be used as a salad dressing, mayonnaise substitute, or base in an infusion with a variety of spices. While this oil does contain 26 percent of one's daily dose of vitamin E, many of the polyphenols and antioxidants that are typically present are lost during the production process of most grapeseed oil products. In a study involving fifty-six participants, about 3 tablespoons of grapeseed oil was added to their daily diet. After three weeks, their HDL cholesterol levels rose by 4 points.

Fourth: Sunflower Seeds and Oil

Refined sunflower oil's smoke point is 450°F, compared to its unrefined counterpart of 225°F, making the refined version perfect for deep-frying, and the unrefined great for dressings. There are a variety of forms of sunflower oil, varying in their polyunsaturated and monounsaturated fats, but all have low amounts of saturated fats. Traditional sunflower oil contains about 68 percent linoleic acid, whereas a newer hybrid version contains 60 percent oleic (a monounsaturated fat). Sunflower oil contains more vitamin E than any other vegetable oil, supplying nearly 40 percent of one's DV, not to mention it is the lowest in saturated fat. Out of three main types of sunflower oils, a variety called NuSun has the lowest concentration of saturated fat. A diet high in oleic sunflower oil and NuSun has been shown to improve an individual's cholesterol profile (boosting HDL cholesterol and lowering LDL), in addition to improving triglyceride levels.

Fifth: Flaxseed Oil

Flaxseed oil, also referred to as linseed oil, contains both omega-3 and omega-6 fatty acids. This clear to yellowish liquid has numerous nonfood applications, such as in paint, wood finishes, and linoleum, and of course is also a nutritious food and dietary supplement. Flaxseed oil contains 26 percent of one's daily dose of vitamin E, which, as in walnuts, comes in the gamma-tocopherol form! Studies have found that fats in flax may reduce heart disease through several mechanisms, including making platelets less sticky, reducing inflammation, promoting blood vessel health, and reducing risk of arrhythmia, as well as having other health benefits.

Sixth: Soybeans

Soy again makes the list, this time for being an excellent source of PUFAs (see page 291 for the broader profile of this healthy legume). A Chinese study found that soybeans added to the diets of healthy volunteers improved immune and brain function.

Seventh: Corn Oil

Besides being an excellent source of polyunsaturated fats, corn oil is also rich in plant phytosterols. Subjects who consumed commercial corn oil versus sterol-free corn oil had substantially lower cholesterol levels, which were attributed to the effects of phytosterols more than to the effects of the polyunsaturates in corn oil.

TOP 7 SOURCES OF OMEGA-3 FATS

SNEAK-A-PEEK: RANKINGS AT A GLANCE

Ranking	Food	Serving	Amount (mg)
First Place	Flaxseed oil	1 tablespoon	7,258
	Flaxseeds (whole)	2 tablespoons	4,700
First Runner-Up	Chia seeds (dried)	1 ounce	5,055
Second Runner-Up	Walnuts	1 ounce	2,542
Fourth	Salmon, farmed* (cooked)	3 ounces	2,150
	Wild, Atlantic* (cooked)	3 ounces	1,730
Fifth	Soybeans (roasted)	¾ cup	1,886
Sixth	Herring* (cooked or pickled)	3 ounces	1,884
Seventh	Sablefish* (cooked)	3 ounces	1,807

*Asterisked foods are sources of long-chain omega-3 fat, which is the preferred source for absorption. Short-chain omega-3 fats (ALA) must be converted into the long-chain form for absorption and it is estimated that, at best, your body will only convert 25 percent of those into the long-chain form.

SOURCES: USDA National Nutrient Database for Standard Reference, Release 24; U.S. Department of Agriculture, Agricultural Research Service, 2011.

Honorable mentions: Anchovies, mackerel, bluefin tuna, white fish

Best food groups: Fatty fish, soy, nuts and seeds, fortified foods

What are omega-3 fats and why are they so important? Omega-3 fatty acids belong to the polyunsaturated fatty acids family. There are three main types of omega-3 fats in the human diet: alpha-linolenic acid (ALA), eicosapentaenoic acid (EPA), and docosahexaenoic acid (DHA). Although ALA can be converted into EPA and DHA, the body is rather inefficient at this process, particularly when levels of omega-6 fatty acids (linoleic acid) are too high compared to omega-3s. EPA and DHA are derived mainly from fish; ALA, mostly from plants. The standard American diet (SAD) supplies ten times as many omega-6s than omega-3s. Most health experts agree that we should consume more omega-3s and less omega-6s for optimal health.

DHA is the major polyunsaturated fatty acid found in the brain and helps with signaling messages to different areas in the brain. It is vital for the developing brains of children. In a study, breast-fed infants had better neurodevelopment function when compared to formula-fed infants, which is attributed to breast milk's having significantly more DHA than formula milk. That is why infant formula is now fortified with DHA. DHA also helps the body respond to inflammation in the brain and helps reduce inflammation brought about by reductions in blood flow.

Did you know? Omega-3 fats have been found to help reduce overall inflammation throughout the body; prevent blood clots by making platelets less sticky; lower triglycerides; reduce joint tenderness; reduce all-cause mortality (any cause of death), cardiac death, and heart attacks; stabilize normal heart rate and improve blood flow to the heart; and fight depression.

How much? The adequate intake for ALA is 1.1 to 1.6 g per day; and for linoleic acid (LA), 11 to 17 g per day for adults. Adequate intakes have not been established for EPA and DHA; however, depending on the health authority you trust, recommendations for these fatty acids range from 0.11

(Institutes of Medicine) to 1.5 grams per day (British Nutrition Foundation Task Force).

Too much! Side effects associated with consuming omega-3 fats from fish oil are typically gastrointestinal in nature, including diarrhea and fishy belches. Additionally, those who are taking medications to prevent blood clots may find too high an omega-3 fat intake may make them susceptible to more bruising and bleeding.

Supplement it? Omega-3 fat supplements can be purchased in capsule, chewable, and liquid from a variety of sources, including fish oil, krill oil, flaxseed oil, and hemp seed oil.

First Place: Flaxseed Oil and Flaxseeds

Turn to page 288 for more about this remarkable little seed. Besides being the best source of omega-3s, flaxseed is also rich in substances called lignans, which may help fight cancer. In addition, research has shown flax may help combat inflammatory bowel disease, arthritis, and heart disease. A Canadian study found that flaxseeds fed to mice in a diet that otherwise contained high trans fats helped reduce the amount of atherosclerosis (hardening of the arteries), whereas the mice that were not fed flax had significant progression of atherosclerosis. This effect was attributed mainly to the alpha-linolenic acid content of flax.

First Runner-Up: Chia Seeds

Chia seeds finally have grown in value far beyond being used in making silly-looking chia pets. These seeds come to the table with lots of nutrition—10 g of fiber and 5 g of omega-3s—combined, a heart-healthy powerhouse. In addition, chia seeds are an excellent source of copper, iron, manganese, phosphorus, selenium, and zinc, and a good source of calcium, magnesium, niacin, and thiamine. The research is fairly scant and mixed on the health benefits of chia. However, a randomized study on subjects who were diagnosed with metabolic syndrome, a precursor to heart disease and diabetes, found that those consuming a diet that included soy protein, nopal (prickly pear), oats, and chia seeds experienced decreased triglycerides, C-reactive protein, and insulin and glucose intolerance, compared to the placebo group.

Second Runner-Up: Walnuts

See page 292 for the many healthy benefits of this nut. The U.S. Food and Drug Administration approved one of the first qualified health claims for walnuts in March 2004: "Supportive but not conclusive research shows that eating 1.5 ounces of walnuts per day, as part of a low saturated fat and low cholesterol diet, and not resulting in increased calorie intake, may reduce the risk of coronary heart disease."

Fourth: Salmon

I'm sure it's not too surprising to learn that salmon ranks high in omega-3 content. But what many people are shocked to learn is that farm-raised salmon actually contains more omega-3 than wild salmon does! And unfortunately, many experts in nutrition get this one wrong all the time. The reason this is so: The omega-3 fat content of food created to feed farm-raised salmon can be manipulated to deliver higher levels. Choosing wild salmon for its awesome taste or for ecological reasons is a valid individual choice but *not* for its superiority in omega-3 content. Omega-3s from fish oil have been cited as a treatment for high blood pressure, menstrual pain, asthma, and so forth; it has also been scientifically validated that they have an awesome effect on lowering triglycerides. Studies have also shown that including salmon in your diet, along with fruit, vegetables, whole grains, nuts, and seeds, reduces your risk of cancer, heart attack, stroke, and diabetes. See page 291 for the host of vitamins and minerals that contribute to this positive outcome.

Fifth: Soybeans

So here's the deal. MyPlate.gov considers ¼ cup of dry-roasted soybeans to be a 1-ounce protein equivalent. Because the fish examples I'm using are 3 ounces, I offered ¾ cup of dry roasted soybeans for comparison. Truth be told, ½ cup of soybeans would be more equal in protein quantity to that of

3 ounces of fish or meat. Besides, you are looking at over 600 calories if you were to down ¾ cup of dry-roasted soybeans in a sitting—you might want to spread the wealth over a few snacks or meals if you want to go for it. For those 600-plus calories, you most certainly are getting a nutrient dense food as you will find soybeans are an incredible source of nutrients (see page 291). A 2009 study of over five thousand breast cancer survivors found that soy intake was associated with better outcomes. Those who had the highest intake of whole soy foods had a reduced risk of disease recurrence and lower death rates due to breast cancer.

Sixth: Herring

Herring is actually twice as high in EPA (the heart-healthy omega-3) as salmon; however, salmon is four times higher in DHA (the other heart-healthy omega-3) than herring. Turn to page 288 for more about herring. Fresh fish is noted for delivering the most nutrition, but what about canned and salted fish that have been stored for twelve months? It was noted that during processing and storage, the level of vitamin A and E decreased significantly, whereas there was no loss of vitamin D or omega-3 fats.

Seventh: Sablefish

You may have never heard of sablefish (also known as black cod) but even if you have, it may be unlikely that you've seen it at the local fishery. That's because the majority of what is caught is shipped immediately to

> The sablefish is dark brown to black and pale on the belly and resembles cod, thus the name "black cod."

Japan! These fish dwell at the bottom of the ocean, where they are the top predators and consume a variety of fish and crustaceans, which is reflected in their nutrient composition: Sablefish is an excellent source of niacin, phosphorus, potassium, selenium, and vitamins B_6 and B_{12}, and a good source of iron and magnesium. Their high nutrient and high omega-3 content is reflected in their price, making them the most expensive fish in Alaskan fisheries. Like tuna, sables are predatory fish, so they have much higher mercury content than salmon. Sablefish is in the top eleven fish species that meet the nutritional recommendation of the American Heart Association.

TOP 7 SOURCES OF INSOLUBLE FIBER

SNEAK-A-PEEK: RANKINGS AT A GLANCE

Ranking	Food	Serving	Amount (mg)
First Place	Lentils (cooked)	1 cup	14.5
First Runner-Up	Split peas	1 cup	14.1
Second Runner-Up	Soybeans (roasted)	¾ cup	12.6
Fourth	Wheat bran	1 ounce	11.2
Fifth	Pinto beans (cooked)	1 cup	10.9
Sixth	Chickpeas (cooked)	1 cup	9.84
Seventh	Raspberries	1 cup	9.75

SOURCE: *CRC Handbook of Dietary Fiber in Human Nutrition,* 3rd Edition

Honorable mentions: Sapodillas, figs, elderberries, quinoa, guavas, loganberries, prunes, pumpkin, dates, coconut

Best food groups: Legumes, whole grains, fruits, vegetables

What is insoluble fiber and why is it so important? *Insoluble* means that it does not dissolve in water and consequently is not absorbed into the body. The main types of insoluble fiber are cellulose, hemicellulose, and lignans, which help aid digestion by moving food through the digestive tract and helping stool absorb water. Insoluble fiber provides bulk and softens stool, which helps reduce hemorrhoids and diverticular disease.

Did you know? High-fiber foods contain 5 g or more per serving, with good fiber sources ranging from 2.5 to 4.9 g per serving. Research shows that dietary fiber, particular insoluble fiber derived from whole grains, can help reduce the risk of colorectal cancer by as much as 40 percent. Fiber can be a great aid in weight loss, as it adds volume to food and can extend the time spent chewing on foods; that is, increased volume plus longer chewing time equals satiety (feeling full and satisfied).

How much is enough? The amount of total fiber recommended a day by the Institute of Medicine is 14 g for every 1,000 calories consumed. Another way of looking at it is that women and men under fifty should consume 25 and 38 g of dietary fiber, respectively, and those over 50 should consume 21 and 30 g per day, respectively. The reason for the lesser amount is the assumption that older folks eat fewer calories. Ironically, constipation is often one of the most complained-about gastrointestinal illnesses among those over the age of fifty! To date, there isn't a specific recommendation for just insoluble intake, just an encouragement to eat a variety of foods to meet fiber needs.

Too much! It's a double-edged sword. Not enough insoluble fiber can lead to constipation and too much can cause loose and watery stools. Too much fiber can also increase intestinal gas (flatulence), and cause bloating and abdominal cramps. These feelings will go away over time as either the body adjusts to the new intake of fiber or the amount of fiber is reduced. However, it may not be wise to greatly exceed the dietary recommendations for fiber, as it can reduce the absorption of minerals such as calcium, iron, magnesium, and zinc.

Supplement it? Fiber supplements come in a variety of shapes, sizes, and forms that are typically made from wheat bran, purified cellulose, or powdered psyllium husks. Fiber supplements could have negative interactions with prescribed medications, so getting your fiber from a wide variety of fruits, vegetables, legumes, and whole grains might be the best choice when it comes to increasing fiber intake.

First Place: Lentils

Lentils are an excellent source of fiber, and also contain resistant starch, which may benefit blood glucose regulation and cholesterol management and may help fight colon cancer. In a study of 186 men and women, results revealed that those who ate legumes, such as lentils, had a much lower risk of developing colon polyps, which are associated with the development of colon cancer. See page 289 for more about this value-packed little bean.

First Runner-Up: Split Peas

Be they green or yellow, because of their high fiber content, split peas are great for helping lower cholesterol and manage blood-sugar disorders. A large study that followed more than sixteen thousand middle-aged men found that those who consumed legumes had an 82 percent reduction in risk for coronary heart disease. See page 290 to learn more about the benefits of split peas.

Second Runner-Up: Soybeans

Adult diabetics who were given a dry-roasted soybean supplement had significantly reduced fasting glucose and triglycerides in comparison with the control group. Also, the soybean supplement group showed enhanced antioxidant activity, which may contribute to protection against oxidative damage in type 2 diabetes. See page 291 for the skinny on this high-fiber legume.

Fourth: Wheat Bran

Wheat bran, the outer covering of the wheat kernel, is arguably one of the healthiest by-products in the food industry, yet until this century it was discarded until its dietary benefits were realized. It is now typically made into cereals, bran muffins, and can be used as a supplement to foods such as yogurts, smoothies, salads, or other items, to add crunch and nutrition. Wheat bran is an excellent source of iron, magnesium, niacin, phosphorus, selenium, and zinc, and an excellent source of riboflavin and thiamine. It can be used for a variety of digestive woes from constipation to irritable bowel syndrome and helps waste move through the digestive tract quickly and smoothly. It may also benefit cholesterol, blood pressure, and type 2 diabetes.

Fifth: Pinto Beans

See page 286 for a fuller portrait of this powerful legume. Phenolic acids and flavonols may play important roles on the overall anti-

> *Pinto* means "painted" in Spanish. But when cooked, pinto beans lose their mottled appearance.

oxidant activities of pinto beans; however, these can be significantly reduced in standard cooking methods. Steaming may be a preferred way of cooking pintos after they are soaked.

Sixth: Chickpeas

See page 287 for more about this fiber-rich bean. An Australian study found those subjects who made chickpeas a regular part of their diet ate less processed food and high-calorie snacks

> Chickpeas are the basis of such internationally famous dishes as Middle Eastern hummus, *chana masala* from India, and *panelle* from Sicily.

because they reported that they felt satiated (satisfied). They also reported that their bowel habits were the best when they ate chickpeas.

Seventh: Raspberries

Fiber is not usually the first thing you think of when it comes to the nutritional properties of raspberries, but they do pack a bunch of it! Raspberries provide important anti-inflammatory nutrients called anthocyanins (the pigments in red, purple, and blue fruits), which may help curtail cardiovascular disease and diabetes and improve eyesight and memory. Turn to page 290 for other nutritional information about this fruit.

> The seeds of raspberries are of great interest to the cosmeceutical industry. The oil in raspberry seeds is rich in vitamin E and omega-3 fats, and surprisingly, may help protect skin, as the oil has an SPF (sun protection factor) of 25 to 50.

TOP 7 SOURCES OF SOLUBLE FIBER

SNEAK-A-PEEK: RANKINGS AT A GLANCE

Ranking	Food	Serving	Amount (mg)
First Place	**Soybeans (roasted)**	**¾ cup**	**10.3**
First Runner-Up	**Lima beans (cooked)**	**1 cup**	**7.0**
Second Runner-Up	**Artichokes (cooked)**	**1 cup**	**6.6**
Fourth	Acorn squash (cooked)	1 cup	6.2
Fifth	Sapodillas	1 cup	6.0
Sixth	Kidney beans (cooked)	1 cup	5.7
Seventh	Figs (dried)	½ cup	4.0

SOURCE: *CRC Handbook of Dietary Fiber in Human Nutrition,* 3rd Edition

Honorable mentions: Sorghum, teff, guar gum, oats, beans, psyllium, flax-seeds, prunes, dried peaches

Best food groups: Vegetables, whole grains, fruits

What is soluble fiber and why is it so important? Soluble fiber consists of two main subcategories: pectin and gums (not the chewing kind!). When soluble fiber enters the intestinal tract, it attracts water, forming a gel-like material that lubricates food and slows its passage through the GI tract. This gel substance helps slow down and stabilize the absorption of glucose in the bloodstream, which benefits insulin sensitivity and helps manage or reduce the risk for metabolic syndrome and type 2 diabetes. Soluble fiber also blocks some of the harmful cholesterol's being taken up into the bloodstream that can contribute to inflammatory heart disease.

How much is enough? According to the Institute of Medicine, for every 1,000 calories consumed, the optimal soluble fiber intake for women under the age of fifty should be 5 to 7.5 grams, and for men under the age of fifty, 7.5 to 11.5 grams. Men and women over age fifty should consume 6 to 9 and 4.3 to 6.3 grams, respectively, per 1,000 calories daily.

Too much! Although soluble fiber can help manage healthy cholesterol levels, in theory, too much fiber could cause cholesterol to drop to unsafe levels by binding bile acids, whose job is to help with cholesterol absorption. Considering the average American consumes less than 10 to 15 g of dietary fiber each day, it is probably not a concern for most.

Did you know? When attempting to increase fiber in your diet, always add it gradually over a period of time and drink plenty of water to make it effective. Replacing refined grains with whole grains and increasing fruit and vegetable servings are two of the easiest ways to increase fiber in your diet.

Supplement it? Soluble fiber supplements are sold mainly in the form of psyllium husks, the outer covering of the blond psyllium seed. This is commonly the active ingredient in bulk-forming laxatives, such as Metamucil. Psyllium husks are unique in that they contain both soluble and insoluble properties that can help control blood glucose and lower cholesterol, while providing bowel regularity. In 1998, the U.S. Food and Drug Administration authorized the use of the health claim, "Diets low in saturated fat and cholesterol that include 7 grams of soluble fiber per day from psyllium may reduce the risk of heart disease by lowering cholesterol." Psyllium husks are sold in powder and pill form.

First Place: Soybeans

This little bean that could delivers both an amazing amount of insoluble fiber *plus* the highest source of soluble fiber all at the same time! Regular soybeans have, on average, 5 to 6 g of soluble fiber per cup, and roasting them removes the water content and almost doubles the fiber content. See page 291 for the many other beneficial ingredients of soy. Soy protein alone may not be effective in helping to fight heart disease. Whole soy foods, especially fermented soy foods such as miso and tempeh, contain probiotics that have been found to be effective for lowering cholesterol.

First Runner-Up: Lima Beans

Besides soluble fiber, lima beans are an excellent source of numerous vitamins and minerals (see page 286). Lima beans are a low-glycemic food and have lipid- and blood glucose–lowering properties.

Second Runner-Up: Artichokes

Artichokes are an excellent source of fiber and folate, and a good source of copper, magnesium, manganese, niacin, phosphorus, potassium, and vitamins C and K. An animal study showed that artichoke leaves protect against liver cancer and heart disease.

Fourth: Acorn Squash

The two main squash varieties are winter and summer. Winter squash varieties include acorn, butternut, and spaghetti squash. Acorn squash has the highest fiber content, weighing in at 9 g per cup (cooked), for only 115 calories! Squash is an excellent source of iron, magnesium, manganese, thiamine, and vitamins A, B_6, and C; and good source of niacin, pantothenic acid, phosphorus, and potassium. According to researcher Dr. Barbara Rolls, foods that

> Officially, squash is a fruit, not a vegetable. Many parts of the plant are edible, including the seeds, leaves, tendrils, shoots, and flowers.

have high water weight and are high in fiber, such as squash, may aid in weight management. High-carotenoid-content foods such as squash also have been found to reduce the incidence of certain types of cancer.

Fifth: Sapodillas

The sapodilla is a tropical fruit believed to have originated from the Yucatán and other parts of southern Mexico. Sapodillas are rich in tannins (proanthocyanadins). Besides containing soluble fiber, sapodillas are an excellent source of vitamins A and C, and a good source of such minerals as copper, iron, folate, niacin, pantothenic acid, and potassium. Because of their high tannin content, sapodillas make an effective antidiarrheal food.

Sixth: Kidney Beans

Kidney beans are an excellent source of soluble fiber as well as a slew of other nutrients (see page 286). A randomized study of sixty overweight men and women found that those who received an extract of kidney beans had significant decreases in body fat yet maintained lean body weight, compared with those who didn't imbibe the extract.

Seventh: Figs

Dried figs are an excellent source of magnesium and manganese, heart-healthy polyphenols, and soluble fiber, and a good source of calcium, iron, pantothenic acid, phosphorus, thia-

> While most of the world's figs are grown in Turkey and Greece, the United States gets 100 percent of its fresh figs and 98 percent of its dried figs from California.

mine, and vitamin B_6. The polyphenols found in figs were also found in an animal study to have immune boosting and antioxidant properties.

TOP 7 SOURCES OF PHYTOSTEROLS

SNEAK-A-PEEK: RANKINGS AT A GLANCE

Ranking	Food	Serving	Amount (mg)
First Place	Sesame seeds	1 ounce	200
	Sesame oil	1 tablespoon	113
First Runner-Up	Rice bran oil	1 tablespoon	161
Second Runner-Up	Sunflower seeds	¼ cup	150
Fourth	Corn oil	1 tablespoon	132
Fifth	Canola oil	1 tablespoon	94
Sixth	Pistachio nuts	1 ounce	80
Seventh	Wheat germ oil	1 tablespoon	75

SOURCE: USDA National Nutrient Database for Standard Reference, Release 24

Honorable mentions: Peanuts, macadamia nuts, sunflower oil, safflower oil, cottonseed oil, poppy-seed oil, almond oil, apricot kernel oil

Best food groups: Vegetable oils, nuts and seeds, legumes

What are phytosterols and why are they so important? Phytosterols are plants' version of cholesterol; however, instead of clogging up our arteries the way animal cholesterol does, they clean them! Phytosterols are also like fiber, in the sense that they promote the movement of cholesterol down the intestinal tract, preventing or reducing its absorption. Think of it as a game of musical chairs: If there are only ten seats for ten molecules of cholesterol, then all get a seat and are transported into the body. But if you add an additional ten molecules of phytosterols, only five molecules of cholesterol get absorbed because the other five seats are taken up by the phytosterols.

Did you know? There are two basic types of phytosterols: plant sterols and stanols. Despite their different names, research indicates that there are no significant differences in their health impact when consumed as part of a low-fat diet.

How much? The U.S. Food and Drug Administration–approved health claim for plant sterol/stanol esters and reduced risk of heart disease is: "Diets low in saturated fat and cholesterol that include at least 1.3 grams of plant sterol esters or 3.4 grams of plant stanol esters, consumed in two meals with other foods, may reduce the risk of heart disease."

Too much! Intakes of plant sterols and stanols in excess of the recommended 2 g per day dose may increase reductions in harmful LDL cholesterol. That sounds like a good thing, but may be a problem if someone has low cholesterol levels. Besides that, there are no other known problems at this time with taking high dosages of plant phytosterols.

Supplement it? The National Cholesterol Education Program guidelines recommend adding 2 g daily of phytosterols to its therapeutic lifestyle changes (TLC) diet for people who do not achieve their treatment targets with diet alone. To achieve this level, inclusion of such foods as margarine-type spreads, orange juice, yogurt and yogurt-based drinks, and dietary supplements have become necessary. A double-blinded, placebo-controlled five-week study demonstrated nearly a 5 percent reduction in cholesterol in participants when a supplement containing 1.8 grams of plant phytosterols was added as part of their TLC diet. (The TLC diet features less than 7 percent of the day's total calories from saturated fat, 25 to 30 percent of the day's total calories from fat, and less than 200 milligrams of dietary cholesterol per day, while limiting sodium intake to 2,400 milligrams per day.)

First Place: Sesame Seeds and Oil

Sesame seeds come in a variety of colors, not just the white seeds we're used to seeing on hamburger buns, and include yellow, red, and black. Sesame seeds are a excellent source of calcium, copper, iron, magnesium, manganese, and a good source of phosphorus, thiamine, vitamin B$_6$, and zinc. Cold-pressed sesame oil is great for deep-frying because of its high smoke point, whereas the dark brown oil is better suited for stir-frying or sauces and dressings. Sesame seeds and their

> The phrase "Open sesame!" is attributed to the sesame seed's magically bursting opening when it reaches maturity.

oil may have other heart-health benefits beyond their phytosterol content. In a small study of hypertensive men who were placed on a daily regimen of a little over an ounce of sesame oil, it was observed for the first time that they had better blood flow through their arteries; furthermore, this effect is sustained with long-term daily use.

First Runner-Up: Rice Bran Oil

Like other nut oils, rice bran oil is extracted from the kernel inside rice. It has a mild, nutty flavor and is a great oil to cook with because it has such a high smoke point—490°F—and a long shelf life. It is an excellent source of vitamin E and contains another antioxidant called gamma-oryzanol, which has been thought to help lower one's risk for heart disease. In addition, rice bran oil has been shown to reduce symptoms of hot flashes among Japanese women.

Second Runner-Up: Sunflower Seeds

The major phytosterol in these nutrient-packed seeds (see page 291 for the full lineup) is beta-sitosterol, which may benefit prostate and heart health.

Fourth: Corn Oil

Sixty-nine percent of national fast-food restaurant chains serve French fries cooked in corn oil. But that may not be such a bad thing: A double-blind, placebo-controlled human study put men on either a diet containing 30 percent fat mainly from corn oil or from a blend of sunflower and olive oils. Researchers found that the vitamin E content of corn oil did a better job of protecting the DNA of cells from mutating into dangerous cancer cells, compared to a diet with sunflower and olive oil. Turn to page 287 for more about corn oil's benefits.

Fifth: Canola Oil

Like corn oil, canola is also a rich source of vitamin E. "Limited and not conclusive scientific evidence suggests that eating about one and a half tablespoons (19 grams) of canola oil daily may reduce the risk of coronary heart disease due to the unsaturated fat content in canola oil. To achieve this possible benefit, canola oil is to replace a similar amount of saturated fat and not increase the total number of calories you eat in a day." See page 286 to read more about canola's high rank among the many cooking oils.

Sixth: Pistachio Nuts

Pistachios have more phytosterols than any other nut! They are an excellent source of copper, manganese, and vitamin B_6, and a good source of fiber, phosphorus, and thiamine. Pistachios contain the highest levels of the eye-health promoting carotenoids lutein and zeaxanthin, gamma-tocopherol, phytosterols, potassium, and vitamin K, of any nuts. James Painter, PhD, RD, at Eastern Illinois University, conducted research with nutrition students from the university. They were offered pistachios as a snack. Whether the nuts were shelled or in-shell, students chose about the same amount. However, because the shells are not eaten, the consumption of in-shell pistachios was actually 50 percent less. Students reported that they were as satisfied with the in-shell variety as they were with the shelled version.

> Pistachios are one of the oldest nuts in existence and are one of the only two nuts mentioned in the Bible (Genesis 43:11; the other is almonds). It is estimated that humans have been eating pistachios in one form or another for at least nine thousand years.

Seventh: Wheat Germ Oil

Wheat germ is the oily component of the wheat kernel. The oil contains high amounts of octacosanol, a plant nutrient found in some vegetable oils, which has been reported to enhance endurance, reaction time, and exercise capacity by increasing oxygen utilization in cells. It has also been associated with reducing cholesterol. A 1-tablespoon serving supplies over 100 percent of the daily value of vitamin E. Dietary advantages aside, application of wheat germ oil has been used to treat various skin conditions, such as eczema and skin rashes, with some success.

Section 2

BEST FOODS FOR WHATEVER AILS YOU

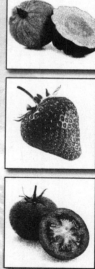

CHAPTER 4
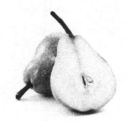
Digest This!

TOP 5 FOODS FOR A SMOOTH MOVE

SNEAK-A-PEEK

Food	Serving
Prunes	½ cup
Lentils (cooked)	1 cup
Psyllium husks	1 tablespoon
Wheat bran	¼ cup
Yogurt	1 cup

Honorable mentions: Kefir, sauerkraut, kimchee, nuts and seeds

Best food groups: Whole grains, fruits, vegetables, fluids, fermented foods

What is constipation and what can be done about it? According to the National Institutes of Health, more than 4 million Americans suffer from chronic constipation each year, which accounts for some 2.5 million doctor's visits. For most, the lack of fiber, activity, or adequate hydration can explain why going to the bathroom can be a painful experience. In other cases, it can be due to stress, ignoring the urge to go, travel, side effects of medication, or a host of underlying medical reasons. So, what exactly is constipation and how will you know if you fit the definition?

Well, for starters, constipation happens as a result of the colon's absorbing too much water, leaving the stool hard and dry, and/or the musculature of the colon is sluggish and weak and doesn't move waste along as rapidly as it should. You know if you're constipated if you . . .

- Strain to go.
- Pass hard, dry, formed stools.
- See bright red blood on the toilet paper (check with your doctor to rule out a more serious condition).
- Take more than a few minutes to do your duty. If you need to take any bound literature in with you, you're bound up!
- Need to take a laxative or enema to go.

Constipation can lead to more than just an inconvenience. Problems associated with chronic constipation include hemorrhoids, anal fissures, prolapsed rectum, fecal impaction, and diverticulosis.

Did you know? An Ohio State study indicates that constipation is on the rise in the United States, and along with it, prescriptions for laxatives. Another unrelated study showed that out of six countries that experience the highest rates of constipation, the United Kingdom led in the use of laxatives as the preferred way of keeping regular versus making a lifestyle change.

Supplement it? Popular OTC supplements include senna leaf and other herbal laxatives, probiotics, magnesium, and fiber supplements. Stimulant laxatives can be habit forming, so discuss with your doctor the best path to address constipation. A registered dietitian can design a dietary program that will help and can advise on what supplements may be the best choice for you.

Prunes

A single serving (four to five) of dried plums, a.k.a. prunes, contains 3 grams of fiber and also includes a variety of nutrients, such as B vitamins, boron, magnesium, and potassium. They are also rich in neochlorogenic and chlorogenic acids, phenolic compounds that may benefit the heart by protecting LDL cholesterol from oxidation. Besides the digestive benefits of fiber, sugar alcohols can also help in laxation by drawing water into the

Shocker Food!

I always feel that water is the unsung hero in this whole constipation business. All you hear is about the importance of fiber, fiber, fiber! But fiber wouldn't be the least bit useful unless it came in contact with water. Fiber takes up fluid and provides bulk in the stool. Your digestive tract senses this and gives you the urge to "go." If water isn't your thing, add flavoring to your water—just be sure not to add a whole bunch of sugary calories. And, yes, tea and coffee will do just fine. For some, exceeding 3 to 4 cups of a caffeinated beverage may have the opposite effect and bind them up. For others, excess caffeine works like a laxative. That said, whenever possible, make your beverage of choice water.

bowel. A serving of dried plums contains about 15 g of the sugar alcohol sorbitol, which may help contribute to the laxative benefit of the fruit. An eight-week, single-blind, randomized crossover study that involved forty subjects compared the digestive effects of a serving of dried plums versus psyllium husks. The number of complete spontaneous bowel movements per week and stool consistency scores improved significantly with dried plums, compared to psyllium.

Lentils

Remember the high ranking of lentils as a tasty means of adding fiber to the diet (see page 127)? This little legume provides an amazing 15 grams of fiber per cup.

Psyllium Husks

Psyllium has been used in traditional medicine throughout the world, mainly as a laxative sold in powder or capsule form. As a bulk-forming laxative, psyllium has excellent water-holding capacity. Psyllium

> Psyllium husk comes from the seed of the plantago ovata plant, an herb grown throughout the world. Most production hails from India.

also has an approved health claim, but for another benefit: "Diets low in saturated fat and cholesterol that include 7 grams of soluble fiber per day from psyllium may reduce the risk of heart disease by lowering cholesterol" (per the FDA).

Wheat Bran

A double-blind, randomized crossover study compared the impact on regularity of three types of dietary fiber, including wheat bran, on fourteen adults. After fourteen days, subjects experienced more frequent bowel movements with all three products; however fecal consistency ratings were highest using wheat bran. See pages 128 and 292 to read more about this grain product.

Yogurt

Many already know that yogurt and other fermented dairy products are loaded with friendly bacteria that the digestive tract just loves. But what many don't know is that regular consumption of fermented dairy products can promote regular, softer bowel movements. You may want to jazz up that yogurt of yours just a bit to get the maximum regularity benefit out of it. A randomized, double-blind crossover study involving forty-three elderly folks with sluggish bowels found that when flaxseeds, prunes, and yogurt were combined, subjects reported that they had more frequent defecation and that their stools were softer and easier to pass. See pages 292 and 289 for more about this nutritious dairy product and its cousin kefir.

HELL BELLY: TOP 6 FOODS TO SOOTHE YOUR STOMACH

SNEAK-A-PEEK

Food	Serving
Apples/Applesauce	1 cup
Artichokes (cooked)	1 cup
Ginger	1 teaspoon
Papaya	1 cup
Peppermint (tea)	1 cup
White or brown rice (cooked)	½ cup

Honorable mentions: Toast, tea, yogurt, gelatin, cardamom, anise, peppermint, turmeric

What causes an upset stomach (indigestion)? *Upset stomach* and *sour stomach* all describe that same horrible feeling that can include any combination of nausea; dull ache; gassiness, bloating, or rumbling; belching or hiccups; heartburn; and a slightly sour taste in the mouth. The most common causes are overindulgence, food poisoning, inadequate hydrochloric acid production, dyspepsia, and believe it or not, even constipation. Most common treatment includes over-the-counter antacids and baking soda. Sometimes not fighting the inevitable (vomiting) is the best course of action.

Nausea is often described as a wave of uneasiness or a queasy feeling that often leads to vomiting. There can be many reasons why someone becomes nauseated: food poisoning (often mistaken as stomach flu), stomach flu, motion sickness, overindulgence in fatty foods, medical problems such as migraine, and hormonal changes caused by pregnancy. Even strong odors and loud noise can trigger nausea. Although not a disease in and of itself, chronic nausea may be an indication of more serious underlying conditions. Nausea can be treated with medication, but natural remedies such as food, herbs, massage, aromatherapy, and other nonpharmacological interventions such as mediation and biofeedback have proven quite successful for occasional nausea.

Did you know? If you have a sensitive stomach, it might be best to avoid certain foods, beverages, and situations that may lead to problems such as fried and other high-fat foods, large meals, alcohol, carbonated beverages, spoiled food, overly spicy dishes, stress, rushing through your meal, and swallowing too much air when you eat (a good reason to not talk while you eat).

Supplement it? Baking soda (sodium bicarbonate) isn't really a dietary supplement, but then again, it's not really a food, either. It is a chemical compound that is very effective for lowering the acid content of the stomach. It is also appears as an ingredient in over-the-counter aids for upset stomachs. Other supplements that are effective are called digestive enzymes. These are typically sold as formulas that contain the essential enzymes that help break down carbohydrates, proteins, and fats. Papaya enzymes, which contain the protein digestive enzyme called papain, come in chewable tablets and can provide relief for an occasional upset stomach.

Apples or Applesauce

If you want something crunchy but not salty to nibble on, apples are your best choice! Applesauce works equally well for indigestion. Choose less tart versions of apples such as Red or Golden Delicious, which are less likely to aggravate your stomach. The fiber in apples helps move offending foods though the digestive tract. Apples are also an excellent source of plant nutrients called polyphenols, which are located mainly in their skin. These polyphenols help protect the gastric mucosa (inside lining) of the stomach, which can become damaged from NSAIDS (anti-inflammatory drugs) and pathogenic bacteria such as *H. pylori,* a major contributor to such hell belly conditions as ulcers.

Artichokes

Along with being nutritious and a good source of fiber (see page 286), artichoke leaves contain plant nutrients that have been found to be beneficial in short- and long-term dyspepsia and gastritis. Research also supports that artichokes are quite helpful in reducing the spasticity that goes along with irritable bowel syndrome (IBS).

Ginger

In natural form as a raw rhizome, ginger may be too strong for your palate, but not to worry! You may find that ginger products such as ginger ale, candied ginger, powdered ginger, and ginger tea are just as effective as chewing on the rhizome itself! Ginger is not rich in any one nutrient but it is packed with the phytochemicals called gingerols, shogaols, and zingerones, which help battle conditions from morning sickness to cancer. This one is time tested! Ginger has been used for the past two thousand years in China to

Shocker Food! ———————————————————

Research has found that those who ate hot peppers as a regular part of their diet had less occurrences of upset stomach than did those who didn't. It may be due to the plant nutrient called capsaicin, found in peppers, which helps soothe discomfort. However, some research supports that adding hot peppers to an already aching belly is probably *not* a good thing to do. So, if you are reading this section, right at this moment, and have an upset stomach, my advice is to skip hot peppers and go directly to the suggestions that follow. And while we are at it, if your tummy problems persist, seek out care from a qualified health professional!

help treat stomach upset and nausea. In a study of subjects with upset stomachs, ginger capsules were found to significantly reduce the time it took for the sour contents of the stomach through the digestive tract. Of course, ginger is also known for stopping nausea dead in its tracks, whether related to pregnancy, chemotherapy, bad food, you name it. There was even a study showing that simply smelling ginger could help reduce the nausea experience after coming out of anesthesia!

Papaya

Papaya is an excellent source of vitamins A and C, and a good source of fiber and folate. It is also rich in the protein digestive enzymes chymopapain and papain. Papaya enzymes are also available in a chewable supplement for the occasional upset tummy. Besides helping proteins digest, papaya has long been known for its anti-inflammatory attributes. A randomized study using a fermented version of papaya for fourteen weeks showed that this fruit was very effective in reducing C-reactive protein and uric acid, both indicators of inflammation.

Peppermint

If you've got that queasy feeling, you can choose among fresh peppermint, or its various forms as a powder, oil or extract, tea, or candy. Try a hot cup of peppermint tea over peppermint hard candies, as sometimes the sugary taste may spur on more queasiness and add calories! Peppermint has been used for thousands of years for medicinal purposes; it helps slow movement of the stomach muscles and/or spasms that contribute to nausea or vomiting; in fact, it helps the entire digestive highway. Research supports its benefits in IBS, too!

> *Warning:* Peppermint can lower pressure on the esophageal sphincters, whose job is to keep the contents of your stomach where they belong— in your stomach! This allows acid to splash back up into the esophagus, creating the burning sensation known as heartburn. If you suffer from chronic heartburn, GERD, or laryngopharyngeal reflux, you may be better off staying away from peppermint of any kind (go instead with ginger; see page 146).

White or Brown Rice

Brown rice is the least allergenic of all the grains and is a good source of magnesium and selenium. Rice is the cornerstone of the BRAT (bananas, rice, applesauce, tea, and toast) diet, which has been Mom's friend for making stomach aches and diarrhea go away (see next discussion for more about the latter). In a study that looked at optimal foods for digestive disorders, rice was found to be an ideal carbohydrate source, for its ease of digestibility and its soothing properties.

> Rice is a staple food for nearly half of the world's population! It is grown on every continent except Antarctica.

TOP 7 FOODS FOR WHEN
YOU'RE ON THE "RUNS"

SNEAK-A-PEEK

Food	Serving
Bananas	1 small
Carob powder	1 tablespoon
Dark chocolate or cocoa	1 ounce
Kefir	1 cup
Miso	1 tablespoon
White rice (cooked)	½ cup
Yogurt	1 cup

Honorable mentions: Applesauce, tea, toast, guavas, psyllium husks

What is diarrhea? Diarrhea is a symptom, not a disease. It is characterized by loose and watery stools occurring once or up to several times within a day. Acute diarrhea is defined as lasting up to several days; periods of diarrhea episodes lasting longer than that are technically referred to as chronic. Immediate health concerns are dehydration and dangerous reduction of electrolytes (such as sodium and potassium) levels, requiring medical intervention if not resolved quickly. The greatest health concerns of chronic diarrhea are malnutrition, poor appetite, and poor nutrient absorption.

The cause of acute diarrhea is often bacterial, viral, or parasitic infection; it is also sometimes attributed to substances in food that are not fully digested. Poor hygiene and living in unsanitary conditions, along with eating tainted foods or beverages, are common causes of infection that lead to acute diarrhea. Sweeteners called sugar alcohols and lactose in milk are examples of substances that some individuals have trouble breaking down. Whereas chronic diarrhea is often a sign that underlying digestive disorders such as irritable bowel syndrome, inflammatory bowel disease, food allergy or intolerance, or other serious conditions may be at play.

Did you know? About 2.5 million children in developing countries that are under the age of five die of the consequences of chronic diarrhea each year, due to *E. coli* and *V. cholera* infections.

Supplements? Probiotics, often found naturally in cultured and fermented foods, such as yogurt, kefir, miso, kimchee, and sauerkraut, have shown some promise in preventing diarrhea, and even greater promise for treating it. Look for probiotic supplements that contain *Lactobacillus* and *Bifidobacterium* strains and the gut-friendly yeast *Saccharomyces boulardii*. Probiotics are available in many forms, such as freeze-dried capsules, liquids, assorted dairy products, and as additions to other food and beverage items.

Psyllium husks are often used in over-the-counter laxative products to promote bowel movements. However, the fiber in psyllium also has the ability to absorb water and form stools.

Severe diarrhea may warrant medical intervention, so always check with a qualified health professional before treating it on your own.

Bananas

Bananas help combat diarrhea by replacing lost potassium, and their soluble fiber from pectin helps absorb liquid in the intestines, to better form and move stool. Bananas also contain inulin, a type of soluble fiber that functions as a prebiotic, promoting the growth of beneficial in the gut. See page 286 for even more about this nutritious fruit.

There are over five hundred types of bananas! The banana tree is not actually a tree, but a huge herb! A banana plant can grow as high as twenty feet tall—as a big as a two-story house! Bananas are thought to be the first fruit to be ever grown on a farm.

Carob Powder

Carob is naturally rich in sucrose (sugar) and a good source of fiber. It is caffeine-free, nonallergenic, and does not contain oxalic acid, a substance known to block calcium absorption. It's a godsend for those who don't tolerate chocolate, as it has a similar flavor. The carob pod has been used for centuries in the Mediterra-nean regions as an effective preventative and treatment of diarrhea. Roasted carob powder added to milk has even been given to infants to stop stubborn diarrhea. (Check with your pediatrician or registered dietitian before trying this remedy with children.)

> Carob, native to the Mediterranean and presently grown in Southern California, is an evergreen tree and part of the legume family. The fruit of carob is a thick and broadly shaped pod. It is grown worldwide for its sweet and nutritious fruit.

Dark Chocolate or Cocoa

Who says that your antidiarrheal remedy can't be fun and taste good? Cacao, or cocoa, as it is more commonly known, is used to make choco-late. It is rich in flavanols, a plant nu-trient that has many health benefits, including the treatment of diarrhea. Foods and beverages that contain fla-vanols, such as tea, grapes, berries, and apples, have been shown to block the loss of electrolytes and water caused by diarrhea. Cocoa contains a variety of vitamins and minerals and may be one of the most antioxidant-rich foods known. See page 154 for more about dark chocolate.

> The cacao tree is thought to have originated in the foothills of the Andes in South America.

Kefir

The "tang" of yogurtlike kefir (pronounced "kee-fur") is caused by naturally occurring lactic acid and minimal amounts of alcohol, created by its fermen-tation. Like yogurt, kefir is naturally rich in calcium and protein and a good source of folate, magnesium, riboflavin, and vitamin B_{12}. A recent review study revealed that probiotics, such as those from kefir, may be protective in preventing antibiotic-associated diarrhea. An active substance in kefir called *kefirin* may have antidiarrheal properties, along with the ability to lower blood pressure, blood glucose, and cholesterol, according to animal research.

This centuries-old drinkable, fermented milk product is thought to have originated when nomadic shepherds carried milk in leather pouches. The warm conditions were ideal to promote fermentation, resulting in a fizzy beverage. Today, kefir is made by fermenting kefir grains that are added to milk and incubated for about 22 hours at 25°C, causing friendly microorganisms to grow in the milk.

Miso

Miso is a traditional Japanese fermented soybean paste. The art of making miso in Asia is akin to wine and cheese making in other parts of the world. Miso can also be produced by fermenting soy, along with grains such as rice, barley, or wheat, with a yeast mold. Although miso contains many different vitamins and minerals, it is not a significant source of any one nutrient, with the exception of sodium. However, miso contains probiotics, and along with other such foods has been shown to prevent antibiotic-associated diarrhea by replacing the lost beneficial bacteria and possibly inhibiting regrowth of pathogenic bacteria.

White Rice

Rice is helpful during bouts of diarrhea because its soft texture, bland taste, and low fiber content are comforting to the digestive system. Turn to page 148 for more about this soothing grain.

Yogurt

Yogurt has less lactose than milk, so many people who are lactose intolerant may still be able to tolerate yogurt. Dairy and nondairy yogurts contain an assortment of probiotics; read the labels. These probiotics have been shown to prevent and treat pediatric diarrhea and prevent antibiotic-associated diarrhea and traveler's diarrhea. See page 292 for the many other nutritional benefits of yogurt.

The discovery of yogurt occurred during the Neolithic era, some ten thousand years ago, in central and western Asia. Primitive methods of storing milk caused unintentional fermentation, thus resulting in yogurt. Yogurt gained international prominence in the early 1900s when a Russian scientist observed that the life span of Bulgarians who consumed large quantities of soured milk averaged eighty-seven years.

CHAPTER 5

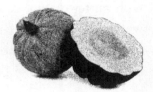

Hearty Foods

PLAQUE ATTACK! TOP 8 FOODS FOR LOWERING CHOLESTEROL

Featuring dietary recommendations from nutrition expert Janet Brill, PhD, RD, LDN, author of *Cholesterol Down: 10 Easy Steps to Lower Your Cholesterol in 4 Weeks—Without Prescription Drugs*

SNEAK-A-PEEK

Food	Serving
Almonds	1 ounce
Apples	1 cup
Flaxseeds	2 tablespoons
Garlic	1 clove
Oatmeal (uncooked)	½ cup
Extra-virgin olive oil	1 tablespoon
Psyllium husks	6 grams
Soybeans (cooked)	1 cup

Honorable mentions: Plant sterol spreads, berries, legumes

Best food groups: Whole grains, berries, legumes

What is cholesterol and why is it important to keep under control? Cholesterol is a waxy substance, produced in the liver that is vital to every cell of every living creature. By the way, plants don't have livers, so there's no

155

cholesterol in them—unless your vegetables are cooked in lard, slathered with butter or sauces, or wrapped in bacon, you never have to worry whether they contain cholesterol or not. Cholesterol is important to have on hand to make hormones, such as testosterone, estrogen, and vitamin D. So if cholesterol is so great, why are we always trying so hard to get rid of it?

Too much cholesterol can have devastating effects on the body, such as hardening of the arteries that contributes to heart disease, high blood pressure, peripheral vascular disease, erectile dysfunction, and the list goes on. According the World Health Organization, one out of every six people in the United States has high cholesterol, and it is estimated that 20 percent of all strokes and 50 percent of heart attacks have been linked to high cholesterol.

Elevated cholesterol can be caused by a variety of factors:

- Family history
- Not exercising
- Smoking
- Being overweight
- Eating too much saturated fat and cholesterol in the diet
- Side effects of medication and/or underlying diseases of the kidney and thyroid
- Hormonal changes with age, such as menopause for women and andropause for men

Optimal cholesterol levels should be lower than 200 mg/dl, but that number doesn't mean that much by itself. Low-density lipoprotein (LDL) cholesterol is often referred to as "bad" cholesterol because of its association with plaque buildup on the walls of arteries, where plaque can restrict blood flow to the heart—or worse yet, a piece of it could break off and lodge in an artery, shutting off blood to the heart or the brain, resulting in a heart attack or stroke. High-density lipoprotein (HDL) has been dubbed "good" or "protective" cholesterol because it helps clear cholesterol from the body. Here is a chart that shows the ranges.

Category	Total Cholesterol (mg/dl)	LDL (mG/dl)	HDL (mg/dl)	Triglycerides (mg/dl)
Low	Less than 100		Less than 40 for men and less than 50 for women	
Desirable/normal/optimal	Less than 200	Less than 100	60 and above	Less than 150
Near optimal		100–129		
Mildly/borderline high	200–239	130–159		150–199
High	240 and above	160–189		200–499
Very high		190 or above		500 or higher

Did you know? Believe it or not, heart disease is the number one killer of women in the United States, and more women have elevated cholesterol than men do! According to the Centers for Disease Control, food is not the only tool in your cholesterol management tool belt. The CDC also suggests that you:

- Engage in daily physical activity—optimally, your exercise routine should be moderate to vigorous in nature for at least thirty minutes every day. This lowers LDL and raises HDL cholesterol (see page 162).
- Although it is good to add cholesterol soaking–up foods to your diet, reducing saturated fat can lower cholesterol even more and protect against plaque formation.
- Talk to your doctor to see whether lipid lowering medications are right for you.

Supplement it? Plant sterols and stanols (collectively known as phytosterols) resemble cholesterol and attach themselves to cholesterol binding sites allowing cholesterol to flush out the digestive tract. You can find phytosterols in plant foods such as fruits, nuts, seeds, and vegetable oils. "Unfortunately, eating lots of plant foods will provide you with only about 300 to 400 mg/day—far less than the recommended amount of 2 to 3 g required to lower LDL cholesterol," says Dr. Janet Brill. "Hence, phytosterols must be taken in supplement form or from the myriad of phytosterol-fortified products on the market, such as margarine spreads, and fortified foods, such as orange juice and yogurt." Phytosterols are sold in supplement form; however, they could possibly lessen the absorption of fat-soluble vitamins. Nutrition experts recommend increasing fruit and vegetable intake and/or to take a multivitamin at the opposite time of day of taking plant sterols.

Shocker Food!

A study featured in *Nutrition Journal* found that female subjects with metabolic syndrome reduced total cholesterol levels and harmful LDL cholesterol after a four-week period of consuming a strawberry-based beverage. David J. A. Jenkins, MD, PhD, has also found that antioxidant levels in strawberries can improve and maintain the effectiveness of cholesterol-lowering diets. The cholesterol-lowering effects of strawberries may be attributed to antioxidants, fiber, or phytochemicals such as elagic acid, found in abundance in this berry. See page 291 for more about strawberries.

The discovery of okra dates back to twelfth-century Ethiopia, where it was a fave of Egyptians. Its popularity grew and okra was even consumed as a coffee substitute. Okra came to the United States via the slave trade and is now most popular in the South as part of Creole and Cajun cooking. Okra is the "quicker picker-upper" when it comes to cholesterol. It's a good source of fiber, most of which is in the soluble form. See page 289 to discover all the nutritional wonders of okra. Dr. Jenkins found that cholesterol-lowering foods, such as okra, that were part of his "portfolio" diet were as effective as statin drugs for lowering cholesterol.

Dr. Brill's daily Rx: Consume 2 to 3 g of phytosterols each day, spread over two meals. "Every food works to lower cholesterol in a specific way; by combining them all, you get an extremely powerful, natural, LDL-lowering approach," says Dr. Brill.

Almonds

Almonds are rich in numerous vitamins and minerals (see page 285) as well as heart-healthy monounsaturated fats, and contain such plant nutrients as phytosterols, proanthocyanins, and flavanols. Almonds lower both total and LDL cholesterol. Scientific evidence suggests, but does not prove, that eating 1.5 ounces per day of nearly any nut, such as almonds, as part of a diet low in saturated fat and cholesterol, may reduce the risk of heart disease.

Apples

Apples are loaded with plant antioxidants. One ingredient in apples, called polyphenols, functions as a powerful antioxidant and prompts the liver to clear LDL cholesterol, limiting plaque buildup. Eating the apple skin ensures the highest level of antioxidant intake. Plus, apples serve up a nice amount of the LDL-cholesterol-lowering soluble fiber called pectin. Find out more about the health benefits of eating apples on page 242.

Flaxseeds

Like walnuts, flaxseeds are a wonderful source of omega-3 fatty acids, a crucial supporting molecule in the anti-inflammation process and fighting plaque buildup. Flaxseeds also contain two other components that target LDL cholesterol specifically: lignans and soluble fiber, the kind that rids your body of cholesterol. A research study that included thirty participants gave either placebo or flaxseed lignans. It demonstrated a statistically significant reduction in cholesterol levels among the flaxseed group that received 100 mg of lignan (one ounce of flaxseeds contains 85 mg of lignan). See page 288 for additional information about the benefits of flax.

Garlic

Although not a whole heck of a lot of other nutrients can be found in garlic, there are ample plant nutrients, such as alliin, allicin, and saponins, which have been found to help lower cholesterol, thin the blood, and boost the immune system at the same time! Garlic lowers LDL by dampening the activity of the main cholesterol-producing enzyme in the liver. Eating as little as a clove a day has been shown to rev up the body's ability to dissolve blood clots, which can precipitate a heart attack by sealing off plaque-filled arteries.

Oatmeal

See page 289 for the nutritional skinny on oats. Cooked oatmeal is an excellent source of soluble fiber, which is composed of beta-glucan, an indigestible polysaccharide shown to help lower cholesterol levels and significantly reduce the risk of cardiovascular disease and stroke. The fiber in oats also binds up bile acids in the intestine so that they are excreted. This forces the liver to make more bile acids to replenish the lost supply, which leads to lower LDL cholesterol. They also contain a powerful, unique antioxidant that counteracts the destructive and atherosclerosis-inducing damage of unstable free radicals.

Extra-Virgin Olive Oil

Extra-virgin olive oil contains two polyphenols, oleuropein and tyrosol, which are known to also protect against lipid oxidation and oxidative stress, not to mention their anti-inflammatory properties. Also, because this oil is so high in monounsaturated fats, it helps maintain a healthy ratio of omega-6 fatty acids to omega-3 fatty acids. See page 289 for more about this super-healthy oil.

Psyllium Husks

Psyllium seed husk is a very rich source of soluble fiber that helps with digestive health and blood sugar control and binds cholesterol and bile acids in the intestine, thus preventing the body from absorbing it. The government's National Cholesterol Education Program advises that all adults consume 10 to 25 grams of soluble fiber per day, but sadly, most get only 3 to 4 grams. Take half your daily dose of psyllium seed husks with breakfast and half with dinner, to avoid overloading your body with fiber, which can cause gas, constipation, or diarrhea. This stuff is very powerful at lowering LDL cholesterol: Just 6 g of this LDL-fighting machine, in conjunction with some of the other foods listed here, can really help to drastically reduce your cholesterol. See page 290 for more about psyllium.

Soybeans

While soy is clearly not a meat or fish, protein-wise it rivals both as a complete source of protein. Soy is a terrific replacement for high-cholesterol and high-saturated-fat meats for those who are keeping an eye on cholesterol. Soy can be found in all sorts of products, including soy flour, tempeh (fermented bean curd), tofu, and a host of meat and milk analogues (fake meats and dairy products). See page 291 for the many benefits of this wonderful bean.

Unfortunately, soy has gotten a bad rap in the press lately, particularly because soy protein contains phytoestrogens—compounds that increase the number and effectiveness of LDL receptors, improving the liver's ability to get rid of cholesterol in your bloodstream but have been under suspicion for stimulating estrogen-driven female reproductive cancers. Don't be misled, as the U.S. government has given soy its stamp of approval as a safe food to help prevent heart disease and leading health experts agree that whole soy foods, consumed in moderation, are safe for the general population and even those with a cancer challenge. Soy is not only a heart-healthy food; it is also associated with reduced risk of cancers. Soy contains isoflavones, hormonelike substances that lower LDL by promoting an increase in uptake of LDL by the liver. Soy also exhibits a strong antioxidant capacity, linked with decreased inflammation of the arteries.

TOP 6 FOODS TO RAISE A LITTLE HDL

Featuring dietary recommendations from nutrition expert Janet Brill, PhD, RD, LDN, author of *Cholesterol Down: 10 Easy Steps to Lower Your Cholesterol in 4 Weeks—Without Prescription Drugs*

SNEAK-A-PEEK

Food	Serving
Avocados	One-fifth
Chocolate	1 ounce
Olive oil	1 tablespoon
Orange juice	1 cup
Pumpkin seeds Pumpkin seed oil	1 ounce 1 tablespoon
Wine	5 ounces

Honorable mentions: Monounsaturated fats, including high-oleic sunflower and safflower oil; alcoholic beverages

What is HDL and why is it important? High-density lipoprotein (HDL) is often referred to as "good" cholesterol, as its job is to shuttle extra cholesterol to the liver for processing, instead of letting it linger in the arteries. HDL levels are inversely related to risk for atherosclerotic disease—meaning the higher, the better. Even if LDL cholesterol levels are below 100 mg/dl—considered a healthy level—also having low levels of HDL can increase the risk of heart disease. According to the National Cholesterol Education Program, people with HDL levels below 40 mg/dL are considered at increased risk for cardiovascular-related diseases.

HDL (mg/dL)	Category
Less than 40 for men and less than 50 for women	Low
60 and above	Desirable/Normal/Optimal

Did you know? While very few foods have been shown to improve HDL levels, some foods and lifestyle choices are known to suppress them.

Dr. Brill recommends you . . .

- **Limit Sugars:** Reduce consumption of foods high in refined sugars and carbohydrates, including refined honey, white breads, and pasta, not to mention those sweetened beverages we love so dearly. Switching to unsweetened iced tea or seltzer water is a great alternative to those beverages.

- **Chew the fat:** People who consume a diet very low in fat may have both low LDL and HDL. Monounsaturated and polyunsaturated fats—found in olive, peanut, and canola oils—tend to improve HDL's anti-inflammatory abilities. Nuts, fish, and other foods containing omega-3 fatty acids are other good choices for improving your LDL-to-HDL cholesterol ratio.

- **Avoid foods that contain saturated and trans fats:** A heart-healthy diet obtains 20 and 35 percent of your total daily calories from fat, with saturated fat being less than 7 percent of your total daily calories.

- **Boost fiber:** Increase the fiber in your breads and pastas by switching to whole-grain varieties.

- **Stop smoking:** If you're a smoker, quitting can bump up your HDL particle levels by up to 10 percent.

- **Shed a few pounds:** Trimming off even a few unwanted pounds can improve your HDL level.

- **Get more active:** Frequent aerobic exercise has been shown to increase HDL cholesterol by as much as 5 percent. Shoot for a goal of exercising for at least thirty minutes or more, at least five days every week. Remember, it's quality over quantity. Better to get that heart rate up for shorter periods of time versus a leisurely saunter!

- **Drink alcohol only in moderation.** Moderate use of alcohol has been linked with higher levels of HDL cholesterol, so if you choose to drink alcohol, do so in moderation. This means no more than one drink a day for women and everyone over age sixty-five, and two drinks a day for men. If you don't drink alcohol, don't start just to try raising your HDL levels. And I already know what some of you guys out there are thinking and the answer is *no*—you can't save all your alcohol servings and have fourteen drinks on Sunday!

Avocados

Hass avocados contain more monounsaturated fats than do the Caribbean and Florida varieties. Avocados provide nearly twenty essential nutrients, including B vitamins, fiber, folic acid, lutein, potassium, and vitamin E. By the way, I think one-fifth of an avocado is a ridiculously low serving size. I eat about half an avocado at a time, which is only 125 calories. If half an avocado was a standard serving size, you'd see more avocado throughout this book!! An animal study showed that rats that ate avocado had about 27 percent lower triglycerides plasma levels and their HDL cholesterol was 17 percent higher, as compared to a control group. In a human study, those subjects with high cholesterol who ate an avocado-enriched diet increased their HDL by 11 percent after only one week. A diet rich in monounsaturated fats, where avocado was the major source of fat consumed (75 percent), was evaluated for its effect on blood lipids. After four weeks, blood tests revealed significantly reduced total cholesterol and LDL cholesterol levels, mild reduction in triglycerides, and significant increases in HDL cholesterol in human subjects.

Chocolate

Share the good news! Dark cocoa (rich in flavanol) raises your HDL and curbs oxidation of LDL cholesterol—that's what we call a "two-for"! Eating a daily sweet treat (just one or two squares (up to 1 ounce) of deep, dark, sinfully rich chocolate will make a significant contribution to the antioxidant potential of your diet. In addition, research shows that dark chocolate reduces inflammation and promotes more relaxed and dilated blood vessels, especially if you're diabetic. See page 174 for more about baking chocolate and cacao.

Olive Oil

The low incidence of cardiovascular disease in countries along the Mediterranean basin is often attributed to olive oil—the mainstay of that regional diet. HDL cholesterol has been shown to increase in Mediterranean diets that include olive oil, especially in comparison to higher-carbohydrate and low-fat diets used to manage cholesterol. One study looked at the effects on children who had elevated cholesterol, when an olive oil–enhanced milk product was used. Those children who consumed the product experienced increases in HDL cholesterol.

Orange Juice

A research study had thirteen women engage in one hour of aerobic exercise three times each week for three months and another thirteen women do the same, except add a little over 2 cups of orange juice each day. At the end of the three-month period, the LDL cholesterol decreased by 15 percent and the HDL cholesterol increased in the experimental group, but no significant change was observed in the control group. In another study, fourteen adults with high cholesterol and thirty-one adults with normal cholesterol consumed a little over 3 cups of orange juice daily for sixty days. Eight control subjects did not consume any orange juice. Orange juice consumption decreased LDL cholesterol in the high-cholesterol group but not in the normal-cholesterol group. HDL cholesterol and triglycerides remained unchanged in both groups; however, the ability of HDL cholesterol to pick up more harmful LDL cholesterol was enhanced. Turn to page 289 for even more advantages of a daily dose of OJ.

Pumpkin Seeds and Oil

The oil from pumpkin seeds is a rich source of phytoestrogens, which help boost HDL cholesterol. An animal study compared intake of corn oil versus canola oil for twelve weeks and found that the subjects who consumed the pumpkin seed oil had lower total cholesterol, LDL cholesterol, and triglycerides, and a much higher HDL cholesterol level than the control group. In a twelve-week, randomized, double-blinded, and placebo-controlled study of postmenopausal women, wheat germ oil was compared to pumpkin seed oil for its effect on raising HDL cholesterol. Each group took 2 g of its assigned oil every day for twelve weeks. The group taking pumpkin seed oil showed a significant increase in HDL and also a decrease in diastolic blood pressure. There was also a significant improvement in the menopausal symptoms, too! For more good news about this flavorful seed, see page 290.

Wine

Red or white? Red wine has *ten times* the polyphenol content of white wine, because when red wine is made, all of the heart-healthy nutrients in the skin and seeds come into contact with the grape juice when it's fermented. In contrast, white wine is made by quickly pressing the juice away from the grape solids. Truth be told, all types of alcohol raise HDL cholesterol. Alcohol increases the transport rate of the major HDL proteins in the liver cells, which help whisk extra LDL cholesterol away. However, red wine stands apart from all other types of alcoholic beverages in its ability to neutralize heart attack risk, due to its polyphenols. See page 292 for the additional health advantages of wine. Remember, though, as with all alcoholic beverages, wine is beneficial for your health only in moderation.

ON THE FAT TRACK: TOP 4 FOODS
THAT LOWER TRIGLYCERIDES

SNEAK-A-PEEK

Food	Serving
Salmon (cooked)	3 ounces
Oats (cooked)	1.5 cups
Psyllium husks	2 teaspoons
Soybeans (cooked)	1 cup

Honorable mention: Sweet potatoes, chia, cocoa

Best food groups: Whole grains; legumes; vegetables; protein such as fish, lean meats, or poultry

Dishonorable **mentions:** All sugars and alcohol! Bummer. Although alcohol raises HDL cholesterol, it can also raise triglycerides.

What are triglycerides and why is it a concern if they are high? Quite simply, triglycerides are fats . . . or more technically, a molecule that contains three fatty acids attached to a glycerol backbone (a fancy term for a molecule that can hold up to three fatty acids).

If you have ever poured oil (pure triglycerides) into vinegar or water, then you can imagine what happens when we consume foods with triglycerides. In our intestines, triglycerides clump up into little balls called micelles. Our body cannot digest or break down the triglycerides in this form, so to break them down further, our liver secretes bile, which breaks up these little fat balls into tinier fat balls. Then a fat digestive enzyme called lipase breaks apart the triglycerides into smaller bits capable of being absorbed into the intestines. Once absorbed, these molecules travel into the bloodstream to fuel our entire body.

While triglycerides play a vital role in keeping us healthy, too much can be a bad thing. Just as with bad cholesterol, having a high level of triglycerides increases your risk of cardiovascular problems. Aim for a fasting level of less than 150 mg/dL.

Level	Triglycerides (mg/dL)
Normal	Less than 150
Borderline high	151–200 mg/dl
High	201–499 mg/dl
Very high	500 mg/dl or higher

Did you know? A small percentage of the population has high triglycerides as a result of a genetic condition whereby small deposits of fat will form under the skin. Numerous mechanisms have been shown to contribute to high triglycerides for the rest of us, but a key component is an increase in the availability of fat in the liver. The liver gets fat from three sources: fat in the diet, carbs in the diet, or circulating free fatty acids from the breakdown of fat in fat cells. (Free fatty acids also prevent glucose from being absorbed in cells of the body and the glucose wanders around aimlessly in the blood, resulting in diabetes.) More common causes for high triglycerides include such medications as tamoxifen, steroids, beta-blockers, diuretics, estrogen, and birth control pills; obesity; poorly controlled diabetes; kidney disease; and excess alcohol intake.

You can reduce triglycerides with medications, as well as by losing weight if overweight, reducing simple sugars, avoiding daily alcohol consumption, and exercising regularly. Portion control is one of the best ways of decreasing both triglycerides and your waistline, which often go hand in hand.

Supplement it? A 2011 study published in the *Journal of Metabolism and Cardiovascular Disease* found that those who consumed 4 g of fish oil per day "experienced significant triglyceride lowering." The American Heart Association supports that people who have high triglycerides take a daily fish oil supplement that supplies 2 to 4 grams of EPA and DHA omega-3 fatty acids. Fish oil therapy has been found to reduce triglycerides by 25 to 50 percent after one month of treatment. Omega-3 fatty acids appear to release the triglycerides from the liver.

Salmon

In a randomized crossover feeding study, twenty-five adults who had normal to mild elevations in their lipids were assigned three different diets: a control diet, a walnut diet (about 1.5 ounces daily), or a salmon diet (twice per week). Total cholesterol and LDL cholesterol were reduced to a greater extent in the walnut diet, but the fish diet produced an 11 percent reduction in triglycerides. Turn to page 291 for the additional benefits of salmon.

Oats

To lower triglycerides and cholesterol, 1½ cups of cooked oatmeal daily is recommended, which supplies 3 grams of soluble fiber. Oatmeal contains beta-glucans, a special type of carbohydrate shown to help lower bad cholesterol as well as triglycerides. Oats in animal, human, and combined studies with other foods, such as soy and chia seed, have demonstrated significant impact on triglycerides. A seven-week randomized, controlled study of 150 men and women with moderately high cholesterol and triglycerides found that in those who consumed four servings per day of high-soluble fiber foods from either oatmeal or psyllium (and had weekly telephone conversations with a personal coach who instructed them on National Cholesterol Education guidelines), total cholesterol decreased by 5.6 percent, LDL cholesterol by 7.1 percent, and triglycerides by 14.2 percent, compared to the control group whose triglycerides decreased by only 1.9 percent. See page 289 for more about the healthy nutrients in oats.

Psyllium

In 2006, the FDA authorized a health claim that psyllium husk and beta-glucan in oats and barley can reduce the risk of heart disease. Many experimental and clinical studies have shown that psyllium lowers cholesterol, controls glucose and insulin, and lowers triglycerides. In a study of type 2 diabetics, the intervention group that consumed psyllium husks for two months had significantly lower triglycerides. Learn more about psyllium on page 290.

Soybeans

Soy and soy protein have been the subject of much research for their ability to reduce cholesterol; however, this legume's impact on triglycerides has not been as well promoted. Several animal and human studies have shown a positive impact on triglycerides. In a study of a cereal bar that contained soy protein rich in isoflavones, twenty-two adults who had elevated cholesterol and triglycerides consumed the bar daily for forty-five days. Triglycerides decreased by 20 percent and protective HDL cholesterol rose by 8 percent without additional diet restrictions in the group that consumed the soy cereal bar.

OFF THE CUFF: TOP 6 FOODS
TO CONTROL BLOOD PRESSURE

SNEAK-A-PEEK

Food	Serving
Almonds	1 ounce
Cocoa	1 ounce
Soybeans (cooked)	1 cup
Spinach	1 cup cooked or 2 cups raw
White beans (cooked)	1 cup
Yogurt and milk	1 cup

Honorable mentions: Tomatoes, kefir, sardines, black beans, orange juice

Best food groups: Low-fat dairy, green- and orange-pigmented vegetables, legumes, fruit

What is high blood pressure and why is it a concern? High blood pressure, also known as hypertension, generally presents without symptoms so it is often referred to as "the silent killer," though there are some who become symptomatic with headaches when their blood pressure is high. Hypertension is a growing health concern, as it is estimated to affect one in three adult Americans (that's 65 million people!), and another 59 million Americans have pre–high blood pressure! Unfortunately, this is also an escalating epidemic in today's youth.

The heart has the awesome responsibility of pumping blood throughout the body so it can carry oxygen and vital nutrients to everywhere it is needed. The force of blood going through the vessels can be measured by the pressure it exerts against the endothelium (the inner walls of the arteries)—this is your blood pressure. There are two numbers associated with a blood pressure reading: systolic (the top number) and diastolic (the bottom number). Systolic represents the pressure exerted when the heart squeezes, and diastolic is the pressure when the heart is at rest. The following chart represents normal and hypertensive ranges for systolic and diastolic blood pressure. Also included is the range for a condition called hypotension (low blood pressure), which can be caused by dehydration, side effects of medications, and underlying health conditions.

One contributor to high blood pressure is atherosclerosis (hardening of the arteries), which may be caused by poor diet, inactivity, genetics, and high blood pressure itself. When the opening that blood passes through in the arteries narrows, the heart has to compensate by pumping harder. This becomes a vicious circle because the extra pressure can cause damage to the lining of arteries. The body's response to injury is to patch it up with cholesterol. Each layer that gets patched makes the lumen (diameter) of the artery smaller and smaller, raising the blood pressure higher and higher. Unchecked, this can lead to clogged arteries to the heart (heart disease) and brain (cerebrovascular disease, a.k.a. stroke).

Category	Systolic (top number)		Diastolic (bottom number)
Hypotension (low pressure)	Less than 90	or	Less than 60
Normal	90–120	and	60–80
Prehypertension	120–139	or	80–89
High blood pressure: Stage 1	140–159	or	90–99
High blood pressure: Stage 2	160 or higher	or	100 or higher

Did you know? The good news is most high blood pressure can be reversed through a moderate diet and lifestyle program. Research shows that the DASH diet (Dietary Approaches to Stop Hypertension) is the best-known dietary intervention for treating hypertension. And for many, the DASH diet combined with physical activity and other positive lifestyle choices, such as maintaining a healthy weight, smoking cessation, reducing stress, and getting adequate rest, can be a lifelong alternative to blood pressure medications.

The key nutrients and foods to limit:

- **Cholesterol, and trans and saturated fats:** Saturated fats play a role in raising the cholesterol in your bloodstream. Studies show that replacing bad dietary fats (cholesterol, and trans and saturated and fats) with more mono- and polyunsaturated fats helps decrease blood pressure.

- **Sodium:** In a DASH study referenced by the *Journal of Human Hypertension,* sodium restriction alone accounted for a significant reduction on both systolic and diastolic blood pressure. No more than 1,500 mg daily of sodium is recommended if you have high blood pressure or are at risk for high blood pressure.
- **Alcohol:** Again, the American Heart Association recommends no more than two alcoholic beverages a day for men and one per day for women. Beyond that, alcohol can contribute to high blood pressure.
- **Caffeine:** Studies show increased consumption of caffeine during periods of elevated stress increases blood pressure and the stress hormone cortisol.

The key nutrients and foods to include:

- **Potassium:** A balance between sodium and potassium is essential for signaling the endothelium to widen to accommodate more blood flow. This process, called vasodilation, becomes compromised in hypertension. A high-potassium diet stimulates vasodilation. Studies by the division of cardiology at Stanford University showed blood pressure–lowering effects of potassium in randomized controlled trials. Research has also revealed that the more potassium and less sodium in one's diet, the greater the likelihood that one will maintain normal blood pressure levels. Many fruits, vegetables, fish, and low-fat dairy products are good sources of potassium.
- **Calcium:** Research shows that people with low calcium intake seem to be at increased risk for hypertension and that increasing calcium in the diet tends to lower blood pressure. Calcium-rich foods include low-fat dairy products, green vegetables, soybeans, nuts and seeds, and fish.
- **Magnesium:** This mineral helps in the production of prostaglandin E1, a powerful vasodilator. Magnesium also helps keep sodium, potassium, and calcium balanced within the cells of the body. The best sources of magnesium include beans, nuts, dark green vegetables, poultry, lean meat, and unrefined whole grains.

DASH essentials:

- Fiber (30 g per day)
- Cholesterol (150 mg per day)
- Fruits (4 to 5 servings per day)
- Vegetables (4 to 5 servings per day)
- Whole grains (6 to 8 servings per day)
- Fat-free/low-fat dairy products (2 to 3 servings per day)
- Lean meats, poultry, and fish (6 ounces or less per day)
- Nuts, seeds, and legumes (4 to 5 servings per week)
- Healthy fats (2 to 3 servings per day)
- Sweets (5 or less servings per week)
- Sodium (1,500 mg per day)

Supplement it? Studies have shown that potassium supplementation may lower blood pressure, but it is rarely recommended that anyone consume such products without medical supervision, as high doses of potassium could stop your heart. Two safer alternatives: Nosh on some beet greens and white beans—and see page 96 for more potassium-rich food choices. A study conducted by the Department of Epidemiology at the University of Pittsburgh found that calcium supplementation resulted in a lowering of diastolic blood pressure. A review study found that supplementing with fish oil made modest reductions in systolic blood pressure over a twelve-week period of time.

Shocker Food!

Although high caffeine intake has been linked to hypertension in some individuals, epidemiological studies suggest that decaffeinated black and green tea may reduce the risk of both coronary heart disease and stroke by between 10 and 20 percent. In salt-sensitive animals, epicatechins, a special group of plant nutrients found in green tea, help lower blood pressure. Scientists have found that drinking black tea can help keep blood vessels from constricting. Additionally, flavonoids found in tea have been associated with reduced body weight and abdominal fat, which also helps control blood pressure.

Almonds

Dr. David Jenkins, at the University of Toronto, developer of the "Portfolio" diet in which almonds are an integral part, found that subjects who followed his diet for a year experienced significantly reduced blood pressure and cholesterol which he attributed mostly to almond intake. See page 285 for additional information about this superhealthy nut.

Cocoa

Cocoa, an ancient remedy the Maya recognized, is only now supported by modern scientific research. Many products contain alkalized or "dutched" cocoa powder to give the cocoa a darker color, smoother flavor, and increased solubility. However, this process also depletes the flavanol content and reduces health benefits that can be derived from them. A review of the scientific literature demonstrates strong evidence that cocoa flavanols lower blood pressure, improve vascular endothelial function, and improve poor circulation. More than 250 studies show that natural cocoa and dark chocolate may have properties that contribute to heart health. See page 287 for more about their benefits.

Soybeans

The results from a randomized, controlled trial of 352 adults showed that soy protein added to the diet reduced systolic blood pressure for those diagnosed with prehypertension and stage 1 hypertension. The study also showed that partially replacing refined carbohydrates with soy protein may be helpful in both the prevention and treatment of hypertension. See page 291 to learn more about the many features of soy.

Spinach

In a twenty-year follow-up study of nearly 4,400 men and women, those who consumed more folate-rich foods, such as spinach and other dark, leafy greens, were less likely to have hypertension when they were older. Read more about this vegetable on page 291.

White Beans

Studies show that individuals who consume high-fiber foods, such as beans, tend to have lower blood pressure. One study looked at the effects of magnesium and potassium, something beans have by the boatload, and found that men who consumed such foods had substantially lower risk of stroke. Research from the March issue of the *Journal of Hypertension* shows that adding dietary fiber to the diet was associated with a significant reduction in both systolic and diastolic blood pressure in people with hypertension. Studies by *Nutrition Reviews* show that increasing fiber intake lowers blood pressure and serum cholesterol levels. Learn more about this bean on page 286.

Yogurt

A recent meta-analysis investigating over forty-five thousand subjects found that individuals who consumed more than three servings a day of dairy products, such as yogurt, saw a significant drop in their blood pressure compared to those who consumed less than half a serving a day. See page 292 for numerous other reasons to consume this food.

CHAPTER 6
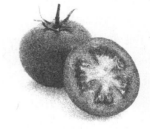

Sugar Blues

DOWN AND OUT: TOP 7 FOODS
FOR RESOLVING HYPOGLYCEMIA

Featuring dietary recommendations from nutrition expert Toby Smithson, RD, LDN, creator of DiabetesEveryDay.com

SNEAK-A-PEEK

Food	Serving
Apricots	8
Fruit juice or soda	½ cup
Glucose tablets Glucose gel Corn syrup	4 1 tablespoon 1 tablespoon
Honey	1 tablespoon
Jelly beans	20 small
Raisins	2 tablespoons
Oranges	1 large

Honorable mentions: Table sugar, jam, gumdrops, hard candy, icing and frosting

What is hypoglycemia? Hypoglycemia, or low blood sugar, occurs when blood levels of glucose fall below 70 mg/dl. The most common cause can be the side effect of drugs used for the treatment of diabetes; however, other medications and health challenges can also lower glucose levels. For diabetics on these medications, hypoglycemia can result from meals or snacks that are too small, delayed, or skipped; increased physical activity; or alcoholic beverages. Symptoms of hypoglycemia include fatigue, dizziness, lightheadedness, headache, irritability, fainting spells, depression, anxiety, cravings for sweets, confusion, night sweats, weakness in the legs, swollen feet, chest tightness, constant hunger, nervous habits, mental disturbances, and insomnia.

TOBY'S TIP

Toby Smithson, RD, CDE, is a spokesperson for the Academy of Nutrition and Dietetics and also a diabetes expert, having managed her own diabetes for the past forty years.

The most effective way to treat hypoglycemia is with glucose tablets or gel. But if the situation isn't urgent, more palatable options, such as hard candy, regular soda, table sugar, honey, or juice work well. Avoid carbohydrates combined with fat or protein—they can slow the absorption of glucose into the blood. When people have low blood sugar, they often feel like eating enormous amounts. It is important to follow the "rule of 15" to avoid a bounce to hyperglycemia.

1. Test your blood sugar.
2. If it is 70mg/dL or below, eat 15 g of a fast-acting carbohydrate source.
3. Test in 15 minutes; if blood sugar is still 70 or below, treat again with 15 g of carbohydrate.

Did you know? Low blood sugar occurs more frequently in people with type 1 diabetes. Almost 26 million children and adults in the United States have diabetes, and it is estimated that 79 million have prediabetes. Complications include heart disease and stroke, high blood pressure, blindness, kidney failure, neuropathy, and amputations. In 2007, the cost of diabetes in the United States was close to $174 billion, including $58 billion for indirect costs, such as disability, work loss, and premature mortality.

Apricots

There are about forty different varieties of apricots—all an excellent source of vitamin A. They are also a good source of fiber, potassium, and vitamin C. Eight dried apricots provide 15 g of carbohydrate. They are easy to carry with you to treat low blood sugar. Apricots are also an excellent source of potassium, which can help with electrolyte balance if someone is perspiring as a side effect of hypoglycemia.

Fruit Juice or Soda

All juices and regular soda contain about the same amount of carbohydrates, but when it comes to juices, not all of them impact blood sugar levels to the same degree. One-half cup of apple, cranberry, orange, or grape juice (most popular juices for raising blood glucose) contains 15 g of carbohydrate, and you can buy juice in convenient aseptic boxes that don't require refrigeration. Read the nutrition labels to determine the correct serving size to obtain 15 g from other juices or sodas.

Glucose Tablets, Gel or Corn Syrup

You won't find these items anywhere else in the book because they have only one purpose and one benefit. If you don't have diabetes or reactive hypoglycemia, there is no reason for adding glucose or corn syrup into your diet. Simply put, glucose tabs and gels contain 100 percent glucose—the fastest solution to raising your blood glucose back to normal. Corn syrup, made from the starch of corn, is 15 to 20 percent dextrose (glucose). It is not as sweet as sugar (sucrose). In fact, it's practically flavorless, but still useful as a sweetening agent in the food industry because it crystallizes less readily than sugar. Three small adult studies have shown that oral glucose is the best treatment for low blood sugar. The American Diabetes Association recommends glucose as the go-to treatment, although the ADA notes that any carbohydrate source may be used. Glucose or sucrose is recommended by both the Canadian Diabetes Association and the International Society for Pediatric and Adolescent Diabetes. Glucose and sucrose were significantly more effective than was fructose at treating hypoglycemia in pediatric diabetics.

Honey

Honey is produced by bees' breaking down the sucrose in plant nectar. The result is a thick syrup that contains glucose, fructose, water, and a minimal amount of assorted nutrients, such as vitamins, minerals, and amino acids, which is absorbed fairly quickly by the bloodstream. One tablespoon contains 17 g of carbohydrate. The color and flavor of honey results from which plant species the nectar was tapped. The darker the honey, the more antioxidants are contained within. The exception to that rule is for light clover honey (which is high in antioxidants) and dark mesquite honey (which is low in antioxidants). The American Diabetes Association recommends administering a tablespoon of honey when symptoms of hypoglycemia strike. Honey contains a one-to-one ratio of glucose to fructose, and although it is absorbed slightly less quickly than table sugar, it is a better choice overall because of its antioxidant content.

Jelly Beans

I never thought I'd have a recommendation for eating candy in any of my books, but here it is! Keep in mind that hypoglycemia can be a killer, so this is sweet emergency medicine we are talking about here! Same deal applies here as with glucose tablets: They

> President Ronald Reagan was known to love jelly beans. In fact, the blueberry Jelly Belly bean was invented for Reagan's 1981 inauguration. The very first jelly bean was developed in the 1800s by an American candy maker.

have a high glycemic index rating and are recommended by the American Diabetes Association as fast-acting sugars to treat hypoglycemia. Although other candies will do the trick too, Toby likes these because they are very portable, not messy, and easy to divide into doses—they come in a wide variety of flavors, too. Have a few but be careful not to go overboard because they are very effective at keeping up your blood sugar!

Raisins

Raisins have a moderate amount of fiber, but are concentrated enough in sugar to override fiber's ability to slow sugar absorption. They are recommended by the American Diabetes Association to raise blood sugar and are convenient and inexpensive, which makes them a good choice for people prone to acute hypoglycemic episodes. As an alternative to raisins, Toby likes to use frozen grapes—seventeen grapes is a 15 g carbohydrate

> About 99.5 percent of the raisins eaten by Americans and 40 percent consumed around the world are grown in California.

serving. "I purchase grapes when in season and then freeze them in baggies based on a serving size. Depending on how low a blood sugar reading [is], I can easily adjust how many grapes to munch, so I don't end up with a higher blood sugar reading."

Oranges and Orange Juice

One medium-size orange is a 15 g serving of carbohydrate. Toby likes oranges because they are affordable, easy to find, and able to be kept in the car or purse, which makes them a convenient snack to prevent low blood sugar episodes. Canned oranges and orange juice are other quick-sugar options. See pages 44 and 165 for more about the benefits of orange juice.

SUGAR RUSH: TOP 7 FOODS FOR CONTROLLING BLOOD SUGAR

Featuring dietary recommendations from nutrition expert Toby Smithson, RD, LDN, creator of DiabetesEveryDay.com.

SNEAK-A-PEEK

Food	Serving
Barley (cooked)	½ cup
Beans (cooked)	1 cup
Nuts	1 ounce
Oats (cooked)	½ cup
Olive oil	1 tablespoon
Wild salmon (cooked)	3 ounces
Greek Yogurt	1 cup

Honorable mentions: Green tea, basil, whole grains, fresh vegetables, sea vegetables, brewer's yeast, and *exercise*

Best food groups: Whole grains, vegetables, legumes, nuts and seeds, low-fat dairy, berries

What is hyperglycemia? Hyperglycemia, or high blood sugar, can wreak havoc in the body, causing permanent damage to tissues and organs. Usually, this condition does not occur in healthy individuals or those who are not diabetic. Unfortunately (or fortunately . . . depending on the way you look at it), many first discover they have diabetes after an abnormally high blood glucose reading.

Blood Sugar by the Numbers	
Fasting blood glucose	**Reading (mg/dl)**
Healthy blood glucose	under 100
Prediabetes	100–125
Diabetes	more than 125*

*The diagnosis of diabetes is often determined by abnormal fasting readings on two separate days. However, your doctor may suggest additional testing, such as an oral glucose tolerance test, and/or having additional blood tests performed. If you suspect you have diabetes, see your doctor.

High blood glucose in those with diabetes can be caused by a number of factors, including excess carbohydrate intake, missed timing or amount of insulin/blood glucose-lowering medication, infection or other illness, stress, inactivity or too much strenuous activity. Apart from diabetes, other conditions and situations that can cause high blood sugar, including medicines such as steroids, severe stress, growth hormone abnormalities, heart attack, stroke, and Cushing's syndrome. Symptoms of hyperglycemia often include frequent thirst not satisfied by drinking fluids, headache, difficulty concentrating, blurred vision, frequent urination, fatigue, and weight loss.

Untreated hyperglycemia may lead to a condition called ketoacidosis, or worse yet, a diabetic coma. Prolonged hyperglycemia can cause chronic vaginal and skin infections; slow-healing of cuts and sores, leading to possible amputation of extremities; decreased or loss of vision; temporary or permanent nerve damage (neuropathy); and stomach and intestinal problems.

Did you know? As little as one single exercise session (regardless of intensity) was shown to improve blood glucose for that day and the next. Physical activity, a healthy diet, and proper medical care are the best ways to control blood glucose.

Barley

The most common form of barley is pearled barley—referring to what is left over after removing the inedible coarse outer layer, or hull. However, hull-free varieties are now being grown. Besides being an excellent source of fiber, manganese, selenium, and thiamine, and a good source of copper, magnesium, niacin, and phosphorus, barley is the richest grain source of the mineral chromium which also aids in controlling blood glucose. Of all the grains, barley has the most cholesterol-lowering beta-glucans content, and it is a great source of both insoluble fiber and soluble fiber, which help block the cholesterol absorption that contributes to plaque formation in the arteries, a condition often afflicting many with poorly controlled diabetes. A meal containing barley significantly improved postmeal insulin response in obese women at risk for insulin resistance. Although barley is high in carbohydrates, it has been shown to help improve insulin sensitivity and provides better glucose control.

Beans

Beans are digested slowly, encouraging a very gradual rise in blood sugar levels. A low-glycemic index diet that includes beans has been shown to reduce hyperglycemia in children with type 1 diabetes. Soybeans contain isoflavones that can help control insulin-independent diabetes mellitus. Turn to page 291 to read more about the advantages of soy.

Nuts

All types of nuts play a positive role in promoting good health and helping to control blood glucose. Tree nuts are a good source of B vitamins, fiber, iron, protein, and zinc. They are also a great source of monounsaturated and polyunsaturated fat and are low in saturated fat. Nuts lower blood pressure, reduce inflammation, and keep you feeling full and satisfied, aiding in weight management. Specifically, consumption of almonds has been shown to decrease high blood glucose after meals, improve insulin production, and reduce oxidative damage in the body and minimize fluctuations in blood sugar levels; walnut studies have indicated improvement in blood flow, weight loss, and weight maintenance, regulating insulin levels, and improvements in blood lipid levels in adults with type 2 diabetes.

A legume often misidentified as a nut is of tremendous benefit toward balancing out blood sugar: A daily dose of peanuts (1.5 ounces per day) reduces the risk of diabetes by one quarter! See page 289 for more about this nifty bean.

Oats

The beta-glucan found in oats has been shown to slow postmeal blood glucose levels and improve insulin responses. Studies have revealed that oats, as well as oat extracts containing soluble fiber, control glucose, insulin, and glucagon response when carbohydrates are consumed. Oats also help control appetite by making you feel full longer. A study of uncontrolled diabetics found that eating oatmeal everyday reduced their insulin needs by nearly 40 percent! Read more about the many benefits of oats on page 289.

Olive Oil

An excess of fat in the diet of diabetics usually spells trouble. However, foods containing monounsaturated fat have been shown to decrease the rates of metabolic syndrome, a condition that occurs before prediabetes.

The use of olive oil has been shown to decrease the risk of developing type 2 diabetes, and reduces the incidence of heart disease by half. See page 116 for a fuller profile of this wondrous oil, the boon of the Mediterranean diet.

> Olive oil was introduced to Americans in the 1700s when Franciscan missionaries come to settle in California brought olive trees with them.

Wild Salmon

Wild salmon is one of the highest food sources of vitamin D, an excellent source of niacin and protein, and a good source of omega-3 fatty acids, selenium, and vitamin B. Deficiency in vitamin D is related to many diseases including osteoporosis, cardiovascular disease, and multiple sclerosis, and has been found to be associated with development of type 1 and type 2 diabetes and metabolic syndrome. Vitamin D plays a role in how much insulin the body makes. Any kind of salmon is also a significant source of omega-3 fatty acids, which reduce chronic inflammation and insulin resistance. "This low in saturated fat and high protein food source helps keep you full but doesn't clog your arteries," says Toby. You can read more about salmon on page 291.

Greek Yogurt

Researchers have recently discovered that a compound called trans-palmitoleic acid, which is found in dairy products, can decrease the risk of diabetes. People who had the highest levels of trans-palmitoleic acid reduced their risk of developing type 2 diabetes by more than half compared to those having the lowest levels. Trans-palmitoleic acid is present in all dairy products, but the bonus of using low-fat Greek yogurt is the staying power of protein—twice that of regular yogurt—to keep you full and satisfied. For more about yogurt, turn to page 292.

CHAPTER 7
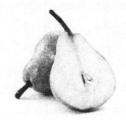

Oral Majority

TAKE MY BREATH AWAY:
TOP 7 FOODS FOR STOPPING BAD BREATH

SNEAK-A-PEEK

Food	Serving
Apples	1 small
Cherries	1 cup
Lettuce	2 cups
Milk	1 cup
Pears	1 medium
Green tea	1 cup
Yogurt	1 cup

Honorable mentions: Water, prunes, peaches, plums, apricots, berries, bananas, honey, agave, avocados, peppermint, gum, cinnamon, basil, mushrooms, cardamom, lettuce, endive, eggplants, cranberries

*Dis*honorable mentions: Smoking, alcohol, spicy foods, sugar, coffee, black tea, onions, garlic

What is bad breath? Eating foods that have a strong odor associated with them certainly can cause halitosis, or bad breath. But the driving force behind chronic halitosis is often poor dental care. Neglecting to floss and brush your teeth allows food particles to remain and feed odor-causing bacteria in the mouth. If dental hygiene is neglected for a long time, it can cause gum disease, which occurs when plaque builds up on the teeth. Bacterial overgrowth can also cause yeast infections in the mouth and cavities. Simply by brushing your teeth and tongue twice a day and flossing once a day, you can do a great deal in reducing foul mouth odor. Semi-annual teeth cleanings and dental exams to rule out tooth decay and gum disease are essential for sweet-smelling breath.

Got that covered? If you still have offensive breath, look into these factors for the root cause: smoking; drinking alcohol; having a dry mouth or dehydration; not eating for long periods of time; certain medications; a low-carb/high-protein diet; or having health problems, especially digestive woes such as heartburn, reflux, or constipation. Foods with strong odors may need to pass through the body completely for the bad breath to end; however some foods' odor, such as that of garlic, may even be detected seeping through the skin!

Did you know? It's estimated that 65 percent of Americans have bad breath. About a billion dollars a year is spent on such products as gum and mints, which mask but do not eliminate the causes of bad breath.

Apples

In a study evaluating a variety of different fruits' and vegetables' affect on combating garlic breath, eating an apple significantly reduced garlic odor. The vitamin C, and saliva produced by eating an apple, also may have a positive effect on keeping breath smelling fresh. Read more about this healthy fruit on page 242.

> Apple-bobbing began as a Celtic New Year's tradition to predict one's future spouse.

Cherries

Although there are several types of cherries, they fall into one of two categories: sweet or tart. Cherries are a good source of fiber and vitamin C. The antioxidants in cherries help keep inflammation in check, and it is thought that some of the phytonutrients in this fruit, such as anthocyanins, which give cherries their wonderful red color, help remove the odor of methyl mercaptan, the colorless gas released in decaying organic matter and garlic.

Lettuce

Often thought as being the least nutritious vegetable, lettuce may be one of the easiest and most effective tools you have at your fingertips to fight dragon breath and stop friends and family from saying, "Let-tuce back away from *YOU!*" Romaine, an example of a nutritionally superior lettuce variety, contains more vitamin A and C than

> Most of the lettuce served and eaten in the United States comes from the New York variety or Imperial strain, which is very similar to but wrongly called iceberg lettuce. Iceberg lettuce, in fact, has red-tinged leaves.

do most other varieties and also the plant nutrients lutein and zeaxanthin, which promote eye and other areas of health. Lettuce has shown high activity in human studies for removing the odor of methyl mercaptan.

Milk

Studies have demonstrated that cow's milk reduced the odor of many malodorous substances, such as thiols, sulfides, and disulfides, commonly found in the Allium family (garlic, onions, leeks, and chives). Whole milk seemed

> The oldest evidence of milking animals was found in a cave painting series in the Libyan Sahara. Milking and cheese making dates back to 5000 BC.

to be a little more effective than the nonfat variety in this regard. See page 289 to learn why else milk is good for you.

Pears

Pears taste much better when they ripen off the tree rather than on! Like apples, pears are an excellent source of fiber, particularly insoluble fibers called cellulose, hemicellulose, lignan, and pectin, which research supports as fighting heart disease, diabetes, and cancer. They are also a good source of vitamin C. Pears were found to be effective for reducing phlegm, a source of bad breath. Also, unripe pears significantly reduced bad breath from eating garlic in a study.

Green Tea

Both green and black tea come from the same plant, *Camellia sinensis*. However, green tea is a richer source of epigallocatechin-3-gallate (ECGC), the subject of much research for its free radical–scavenging and cancer-fighting properties. The polyphenols in green tea fight bacteria that lead to dental caries and neutralize odor-causing sulfur compounds from other foods and bad bacteria.

Yogurt

A daily dose of yogurt reduced malodorous hydrogen sulfide in a study. This may be due to certain strains of friendly bacteria, such as *Streptococcus thermophilus* and *Lactobacillus bulgaricus*, which compete for growth with bad bacteria that contribute to bad breath. See page 292 for the skinny on the many other properties of this fermented food.

TOOTH OR CONSEQUENCES: TOP 7 FOODS FOR FIGHTING CAVITIES

Featuring expert nutrition advice from Toby Amidor, MS, RD, a food and nutrition consultant and owner of TobyAmidorNutrition.com

SNEAK-A-PEEK

Food	Serving
Apples	1 small or ½ large
Cheese	1.5 ounces hard cheese, ⅓ cup shredded
Cocoa	1 tablespoon
Cranberries	1 cup
Peanuts	1 ounce
Black tea	1 cup
Yogurt or kefir	1 cup

Honorable mentions: Dairy products, whole grains, berries, nuts and seeds, fresh fruit, vegetables such as celery and carrots, salmon and other fatty fish, dark chocolate, honey, licorice, the sweetener xylitol

What are dental caries? Dental caries, cavities, or tooth decay all refer to the same thing—the destruction of tooth enamel. This happens when simple sugars remain on the teeth over time and promote the growth and multiplication of destructive mouth bacteria that erodes tooth enamel. According to the American Dental Association, the good news is tooth decay may be prevented by following these four simple rules: (1) Brush twice daily with a fluoride toothpaste, (2) floss daily, (3) eat nutritious food and limit sugary snacks, and (4) have regular professional cleanings and oral examinations.

Did you know? Cavities are not just for kids! Aging predisposes adults to cavities because of receding gums and an increased incidence and risk for gum disease. This puts adults at risk for tooth plaque, especially for those who are over fifty and who are prone to tooth-root decay. Additionally, the dental fillings get old, too! Fillings you first had in your younger years can weaken, fracture, or leak around the edges as you age. Bacteria can take advantage of these crevices and wham—you've got tooth decay!

Apples

The World Health Organization recommends increasing consumption of fruits and vegetables as a dietary goal for both general and oral health. An apple a day may help keep the dentist's drill away. Crunching apples, rich in fiber, helps keep saliva flowing to clean the teeth, and the flavonoids in apples inhibit bacterial growth in the mouth, as shown by experimental studies in animals and intervention studies.

Cheese

Eating cheese helps improve oral health by preventing loss of minerals in teeth. Also, cheese contains casein, a type of protein that helps with calcium remineralization of enamel on the teeth, which helps counteract the acids that cause tooth decay. And it doesn't have to be a lot of cheese, either. As little as 5 grams of cheese can be effective in reducing dental caries. One of the earliest studies on cavity prevention from cheese was when scientists fed Emmentaler cheese on bread to rats and found decreased prevalence of tooth decay. Read more about the health benefits of cheese on page 287.

Cocoa

What do tea, coffee, and cocoa all have in common? Polyphenols! Yes, these unique plant nutrients play a role in the prevention of cavities because of their ability to fight bacteria. Cocoa polyphenols reduce the formation of acid from *Streptococcus* and *S. sanguinis*—the bad-boy bacteria that produce caustic acid that pokes holes in your teeth. Who'd have thunk it? Now to be clear, we're talking cocoa powder here, *not* a sugary chocolate bar. Cacao bean extract was given via their drinking water to rats that were infected with *Streptococcus* bacteria. Those rats that drank the cocoa extract had a significantly reduced rate of growth of glucosyltransferase, an enzyme that helps plaque adhere to tooth enamel. The end result was far fewer cavities. Turn to page 151 to learn more about the properties of cocoa.

Cranberries

Flavonoids are known for their antimicrobial effects and are believed to help prevent tooth decay. Cranberries, and many other berries, are rich in these compounds and organic acids. The flavonoids in cranberries and blueberries inhibit bacteria from sticking to surfaces (cranberries are often "prescribed" for urinary tract infections because they prevent *E. coli* bacteria from adhering to the bladder wall). A study showed that cranberries decreased the cavity-promoting bacteria found in saliva. Additionally, raw cranberries are a good source of fiber and vitamin C.

Peanuts

Peanuts are one of the least cariogenic (cavity-causing) foods you can eat! Peanuts—which belong to the legume, not nut, family—are an excellent source of manganese and niacin, and a good source of copper, fiber, folate, magnesium, phosphorus, thiamine, vitamin E, and zinc. Peanuts may have an edge over peanut butter. Although both contain the same fiber, scientists think eating foods that require more chewing is what decreases plaque buildup: Crunching on peanuts stimulates and improves the flow of plaque-busting saliva. Away from the mouth, eating peanuts has also been associated with reduced risk of chronic diseases including diabetes, heart disease, gallbladder and colorectal cancer, and obesity.

Black Tea

Drink tea without adding sweeteners, as sugars are known to increase risk of dental caries. If you must, use nonsugar sweeteners, such as stevia, or add traditional sweeteners sparingly. Black, oolong, and green tea drinkers may be protecting their teeth by drinking tea on a regular basis. Flavonols, such as epigallocatechin, are abundant in tea and have been shown to diminish the growth of harmful bacteria. Additionally, tea leaves contain fluoride, a mineral that supports oral health by helping strengthen the mineral composition of teeth. University of Illinois at Chicago researchers found natural chemicals in black tea that inhibit the growth of glucosyl-transferase. Turn to page 173 to read additional reasons to take tea.

TOBY'S TIP

Make your tea with tap water!

Because fluoride is added to many water supplies, cooking with it or using it in your tea of coffee can be helpful to prevent cavities. If you don't have fluoride in your drinking water, you can also find bottled water with added fluoride or you can simply brush with toothpaste containing fluoride.

Yogurt or Kefir

Plain kefir or yogurt, combined with naturally sweet fresh fruit loaded with fiber, acts like a natural toothbrush so sugars don't stick. The trick is to add the fruit yourself, for improved texture and reduced sugar. Yogurt contains calcium and phosphorus, which are two minerals needed to remineralize teeth. Often, these two minerals are removed by the acids in the mouth. A study of 2,058 three-year-olds showed that consuming fermented dairy products was associated with having fewer cavities. Also, adults who drank yogurt, fermented milk, and fermented dairy beverages had pH levels that were less acidic and below the critical level for enamel and corrosion to occur.

GUMS AND AMMUNITION: TOP 7 FOODS FOR FIGHTING GUM DISEASE

Featuring expert nutrition advice from Toby Amidor, MS, RD, a food and nutrition consultant and owner of TobyAmidorNutrition.com

SNEAK-A-PEEK

Food	Serving
Carrot juice	1 cup
Kefir or yogurt	1 cup
Peppers	1 cup
Quinoa (cooked)	½ cup
Salmon (cooked)	3 ounces
Spinach (raw) Spinach (cooked)	2 cups 1 cup
Green tea	1 cup

Honorable mentions: Sweet potatoes, white potatoes, pumpkin, carrots, fatty fish, low-fat and no-sweetener-added dairy, citrus fruit, whole grains, nuts and nut butters, seeds

What is gum disease? Also called periodontal disease, gum disease happens when gums and their supporting tissue become infected and inflamed. This process is created by plaque's accumulating on the teeth and hardening into tartar under the gumline. The first signs of gingivitis, a mild type of gum disease, are bleeding gums even during light tooth brushing. Regular brushing and flossing, plus regular cleaning by a dental hygienist, often do the trick.

Did you know? Many nutrients contribute to oral health. Folate and vitamins A and C help the mucosal and connective tissue develop and repair properly. Calcium, phosphorus, and protein are important components of collagen, teeth, and bone. Omega-3 fatty acids and vitamin D regulate immune function.

Carrot Juice

One might think that because carrot juice is higher in natural sugars, it might spell trouble for both teeth and gums. Not the case! Not surprising, carrot juice is an amazing source of vitamin A, supplying 45,000 IU per cup! Moreover, carrot juice is one of the best sources of beta-carotene—a plant nutrient that turns into retinol, which is the form of vitamin A your body absorbs—followed by pumpkin, sweet potato, carrots, and spinach. Beta-carotene intake is inversely related to severe gum inflammation. See page 287 for the additional nutrients in carrot juice. (Be careful! Although not considered harmful, chronic carrot juice consumption can turn your skin orange. This will go away when you reduce or eliminate drinking carrot juice.)

Kefir or Yogurt

Low-fat kefir is an excellent choice for oral health because of its calcium, lactic acid, low sugar content, probiotics, and vitamin D. Probiotics are known to have many beneficial effects on health. The probiotic *Lactobacillus* that is naturally found in kefir helps prevent periodontal disease. These friendly bacteria secrete such substances as hydrogen peroxide, which kills the bad guys that promote gum disease and plaque. Studies show that those who consume little to no dairy foods have a 20 percent increased risk of developing periodontal disease, compared to those who consume more. Also, people who enjoyed two or more servings each day of fermented dairy items, such as plain yogurt and kefir, were less likely to develop the deep pockets and tooth loss that can occur with gum disease.

Peppers

Peppers, especially red and green bell peppers, are rich in vitamin C. This vitamin's active component, ascorbic acid, is an antioxidant that fights within each cell of the body. An NHANES study showed that there is a significant relationship between ascorbic acid levels and the risk of developing periodontal disease—the lower the levels, the higher the risk. Learn more about peppers on pages 43 and 44.

> The seeds of hot peppers are *not* where the burning sensation comes from. The source of heat is capsaicin, a plant nutrient found in the glands of peppers, with the greatest heat found in the placenta—the part of the pepper that attaches seed to the pod.

Quinoa

Quinoa is a highly nutritious whole grain, providing superior protein. It is also an excellent source of folic acid, magnesium, manganese, and phosphorus, and a good source of copper, fiber, iron, protein, thiamine, and vitamin B_6. Moreover, quinoa is a richer source of calcium, copper, iron, magnesium, manganese, phosphorus, potassium, and zinc than wheat, barley, or corn. Risk for gum disease in men decreases as intake of whole grains increases. One cup of quinoa has over 5 g of dietary fiber, which helps clean food debris from teeth. A low fiber intake is associated with poor blood glucose control, which is a risk factor for gum disease.

Salmon

Salmon is the highest dietary source of vitamin D. Low levels of vitamin D have been related to increased gum bleeding. Learn more about this super nutritious fish on page 291.

Spinach

Toby suggests that spinach may be protective against gum disease because it is rich in vitamins A (carotenoids) and C and contains fiber and folate.

These are all nutrients associated with protection against gum disease. See page 291 for the many more nutrients in this power-packed green.

> Spinach has been used in European cuisine since the fifteenth century, but was not embraced in the United States until the early nineteenth.

Green Tea

Green tea contains catechins that decrease inflammatory response to bacteria that cause gum disease. Catechins have antioxidant, antimicrobial, articollagenase, and antimutagenic properties that all lend to the treatment of periodontal disease. Learn more about this healthy beverage on page 210.

> Unlike its brother and sister teas—black and oolong—which come from the same plant, green tea is steamed and dried, which retains the color of the original leaf.

CHAPTER 8

Best for Inside and Out

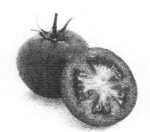

EAT THIS, AGE LESS:
TOP 5 FOODS TO SLOW DOWN AGING

SNEAK-A-PEEK

Food	Serving
Grapes Red wine	1 cup 5 ounces
Olive oil	1 tablespoon
Salmon (cooked)	3 ounces
Soybeans (cooked)	1 cup
Whey	1 ounce

Honorable mentions: Berries, whole grains, yogurt, tea, flaxseeds, avocados

Which foods keep you looking young? There is biological aging and there is chronological aging. Can't do much about the latter, but there are some things you can do to slow down the hands of time's effects on your looks and possibly even reverse damage through good nutrition and healthy living! We'll get to food in a moment, but I want to share some other simple yet effective tips for looking your youngest!

- **Don't smoke:** This is "pedal to the metal" on the aging process. Studies show smoking damages the basic structure of skin cells, which leaves skin looking haggard and leathery.
- **Get plenty of rest:** Besides literally taking years off your life, lack of sleep can make you look older than you really are. Experts suggest at least seven to eight hours of restful sleep.
- **Start sooner than later:** There is a rate of diminishing returns, as noticeable signs of aging start as early as the midtwenties.
- **Sun of a . . . :** Have a love/hate relationship with Mr. Sun. Some exposure is good because it is the richest source for our daily vitamin D supply, which also supports muscles and bones, which in turn hold up your healthy skin. But overexposure can wipe away all the good of the sun, as it can increase chances of melanoma—a deadly form of skin cancer—and ultraviolet light can also permanently damage skin cell DNA and cripple collagen that supports healthy skin cells. Use appropriate skin protection when you think you will be exposed longer than you should be!

Did you know? Out of all the research on foods that have antiaging properties, the consumption of fruit and vegetables offered the greatest breadth of scientific support. University of St. Andrews researchers recently found that the key to a rosy, healthy-looking complexion was ramping up fruit and vegetable intake. Depending on the type and quantity of fruits and vegetables eaten, noticeable improvements could be seen as early as six weeks, when even the skin looked healthier and more attractive: Warmer and more youthful yellow and red hues were accented and cooler colors were more muted with increased fruit and vegetable consumption, mainly because the carotenoids in green, red, yellow, and orange fruits and veggies reflect in the skin's surface when we eat them habitually.

How much do you have to eat for an awesome you? Surprisingly, just three servings of carotenoid-rich produce items such as carrots, yams, spinach, peaches, pumpkin, apricots, watermelon, tomatoes, and pink grapefruits over the six-week period was enough to show noticeable improvement in that study. Not surprisingly, I will encourage you to eat these carotenoid-rich veggies more frequently (like daily!) to improve your skin and everything else underneath it!

Supplement it? Nutrient deficiencies associated with less than optimal health of hair, nails, or skin include protein, zinc, calcium, and iron, B vitamins, such as biotin, and vitamins A and C, and omega-3s. Dietary supplements can provide these nutrients, but first look to optimizing your diet before purchasing these nutrients in supplement form.

Shocker Food! ———————————————

Yes, chocolate once again! Often the very last food that people think of for promoting healthy skin, chocolate has wrongfully been associated with poor skin health, but is now extolled by researchers for its cocoa flavanol content, which offers UV protection. A double-blind study involving thirty healthy volunteers randomly assigned them to consume daily either a high- or ow-flavanol chocolate treat for twelve weeks. The high-flavanol group saw a doubling of UV protection in their skin, compared to those who consumed the low-flavanol. See page 164 for more goodies about adding dark chocolate to your diet.

Another study suggests dried prunes may help reduce skin wrinkles. Talk about food irony!

Grapes and Wine

Red wine has antiaging benefits! Lucky you if you enjoy a glass of red wine every once in a while. Resveratrol, found in the skin of red grapes, is an anti-inflammatory and can help slow the aging process. You can also enjoy the benefits of resveratrol from grape juice and fresh red grapes, too! Resveratrol has been shown in several studies to help protect the skin from UV radiation damage that can lead to not only premature aging but also cancer of the skin and other skin disorders. And eating the entire grape may help skin look younger, too. The seeds of grapes are rich in proanthocyanidins, which have demonstrated strong antioxidant protection against DNA damage to skin cells. See pages 245 and 278 for more about grape juice and wine.

Olive Oil

In a review of many studies that looked at the antiaging benefits of a Mediterranean diet, it was determined that olive oil, because of its phenolic properties, exerted the most effect on preventing age-related diseases. Many of the benefits of the phenolic compounds in olive oil are due to its anti-inflammatory effects. A study found that olive oil is as effective as such over-the-counter medications as Advil for reducing inflammation! Turn to page 289 to read about the many nutritional advantages of olive oil.

Salmon

Salmon, as well as trout, tuna, sardines and mackerel, are great sources of omega-3s, protein, and vitamin B_{12}, all benefiting our ins and outs. Broken and weak nails may be a sign of vitamin B_{12} deficiency, so salmon can be great for combating that symptom—a 3-ounce serving provides 40 percent of the RDA for this vitamin! Additionally, these kinds of fish are lower than other animal proteins in saturated fat and cholesterol, both of which can speed up the aging process! What gives salmon its healthy salmon color is a phytonutrient called astaxanthin, which belongs to the carotenoid family. Research shows this powerful antioxidant fights age-related diseases. Read more about this superhealthy fish on page 291.

Omega-3s play a huge role in reducing internal inflammation, which means better circulation. Low intake and body stores of omega-3 can be evidenced by dry skin or an itchy scalp. About 35 percent of the human brain consists of fatty-acids such as DHA and EPA (kinds of omega-3s), but as the years go by the concentration can decrease! A study found that brains of the elderly contained 22 percent less of these fatty acids than the brains of younger adults.

Soybeans

Soy contains many nutrients that benefit healthy aging from the inside out. One of those substances is called equol, which derived from the soy isoflavone diadzen. As women go through menopause, youthful levels of estrogen drop, and along with them, so do skin, bone density, and the list goes on. In a cell study, equol significantly increased collagen and elastin, and caused significant positive changes in skin antioxidant and antiaging genes. The benefit of soy and the supplement equol may be a safer yet effective alternative to estrogen therapy.

Whey

Whey protein is one of proteins that naturally occur in dairy products such as cottage cheese. It is high in branch-chain amino acids, especially leucine, which is attributed to helping muscles repair and grow. Proteins are the main components of hair, skin, and nails, and most of us get more than enough in our diet. But as we age, the muscles that hold up skin begin to waste away. Consuming high-quality protein may slow down this process. Whey protein was shown to stimulate protein anabolism (muscle growth) independent of physical activity for the elderly. See page 264 for more about whey.

THE BIG HURT: TOP 5 FOODS FOR NUMBING ACHES AND PAINS

SNEAK-A-PEEK

Food	Serving
Cherries	1 cup
Ginger	½ teaspoon
Hot peppers	1 cup
Salmon (cooked)	3 ounces
Tumeric	½ teaspoon

Honorable mentions: Olive oil, berries

What causes pain and how can these foods help? We are a nation in a lot of pain. Millions of Americans use prescription and nonprescription drugs daily in an effort to control it. In 2008, nearly 75 percent of all prescription drug overdoses in the United States were caused by pain-relieving drugs. Much of this pain is related to the consequences of lifestyle choices, such as overeating and inactivity that lead to painful joint and muscle pain and also digestive challenges that can cause pain. Inflammation targets pain receptors and set them ablaze. This list of top-researched pain-relieving foods are rich in nutrients that help reduce inflammation and pain—but, of course, seek your doctor's advice for the best path for controlling and hopefully eliminating what ails you.

Did you know? A certain group of vegetables called nightshades could be painful to swallow, especially for osteoarthritis and gout sufferers. A plant chemical called solanine has been found to contribute to arthritic pain, but for only those who may have sensitivity to it. Members of the nightshade group include tomatoes, potatoes (not sweet potatos or yams), eggplants, and peppers (not the black or white seasoning varieties). The good news is if you are someone who suspects that they have sensitivity to solanine, you should see a difference in one to two weeks of abstaining from nightshades. If you don't respond, you can welcome nightshades back with open mouth!

Supplement it? Some research supports that the following dietary supplements may offer pain relief:

- Omega-3 fats (reduce inflammation)
- Glucosamine sulfate (for painful joints)
- Vitamin D (bolsters bone health); many studies correlate low levels of vitamin D with pain
- S-adenosyl-L-methionine (outside the USA, a prescribed drug for depression and osteoarthritis)
- Cayenne pepper (relieves topical pain and reduces inflammation)
- Alpha lipoic acid (reduced nerve pain, a.k.a. neuropathy)
- Methylsulfonylmethane (benefits osteoarthritis)
- Bromelain (an anti-inflammatory)

Cherries

Packed with pure goodness (see page 243), cherries have been found to have pain-reducing effects similar to those of anti-inflammatory drugs such as aspirin. A recent study published in the *Journal of the International Society of Sports Nutrition* found that consuming tart cherry juice before long-distance running can reduce postrun muscle pain. Several studies support the pain-relieving effects in joints, too!

Ginger

Ginger is loaded with powerful antioxidants, such as shogaols, zingerones, and gingerols, which are all effective anti-inflammatories. As reported in the *Journal of Pain*, a randomized, double-blind, placebo-controlled study found that subjects who either ate about ½ teaspoon of raw or cooked ginger for eleven days prior to muscle pain from exercise saw pain reduced within 24 hours, compared to the control group. In another related study, ginger was not effective for reducing pain when it was taken twenty-four to forty-eight hours *after* exercise. The study's authors emphasized the importance of consuming ginger daily for maximum pain relief. See page 146 to read more about this healthy rhizome.

Hot Peppers

Why would something that causes pain to the tongue, or God forbid, touches any of your mucous membranes, be helpful in stopping pain anywhere else? Well, for starters, hot peppers are extremely rich in vitamin C, which helps repair wounded tissue that causes pain. This nightshade contains an abundance of phytochemicals that reduce pain-causing inflammation, such as flavonoids and capsaicinoids, including capsaicin. Capsaicin has long been used externally for pain relief as an ingredient in topical salves and dermal patches, but what about its effectiveness internally? A randomized, double-blinded study of thirty patients with chronic dyspepsia (upset stomach) found that those who ingested about ½ teaspoon of red pepper (2.5 g) daily for five weeks had 60 percent reduction in reports of stomach pain, fullness, and nausea, compared to the placebo group that experienced a 30 percent reduction of complaints. Long-term ingestion of hot chiles was found to improve dyspepsia and GERD symptoms in small randomized, controlled studies. Read more about the benefits of hot peppers on page 147.

Salmon

At this point, you should know that salmon is one of the best fish sources of omega-3s. Its omega-3 and vitamin D have been shown in study after study to help with aches and prevent arthritis and joint soreness. Omega-3s help reduce the production of inflammatory cytokines and enzymes that cause painful joints, muscles, and nerve endings. Clinical studies have shown that intake of omega-3 fats found in such foods as salmon result in reduction in pain associated with arthritis, dysmenorrhea (painful menstrual cramps), inflammatory bowel disease, and neuropathy (nerve pain). If you missed the full scoop on salmon's numerous nutrients, turn to page 291.

Turmeric

Turmeric contains iron, manganese, potassium, and vitamins B_6 and C; however, you would need to consume quite a bit to see any appreciable amount of those nutrients. But as with most therapeutic herbs and spices, its phytonutrients are the stars: Turmeric is loaded with pain- and inflammation-fighting curcumin. Several animal and human studies show that the curcumin in turmeric is an effective pain reliever; for example, a double-blind placebo-controlled study found that this spice was effective for relieving postsurgical pain and fatigue.

FLU FIGHTERS: TOP 5 FOODS TO BATTLE COLD AND FLU

SNEAK-A-PEEK

Food	Serving
Apples	1 small
Chicken soup	1 cup
Garlic	1 clove
Elderberries	1 cup
Green tea	1 cup

Honorable mentions: Turmeric, sweet potatoes, papayas

What are the common cold and the flu? The common cold is caused by a virus in the nose and throat area, and may include the bronchial tubes and sinuses. The cold may last from a few days to a few weeks and can lead to a more serious problem, such as a sinus infection, middle ear infection, bronchitis, or pneumonia. Symptoms usually include sore throat, sneezing, runny nose, headache, and exhaustion. Treatment includes rest, fluids, and over-the-counter remedies such as analgesics, antihistamines, and decongestants. Hand washing is one of the most effective preventive measures from spreading the common cold.

According to the CDC, flu kills as many as thirty-six thousand people each year. There are three basic types of influenza viruses: A, B, and C. Human influenza A and B viruses run rampant every winter in the United States. Influenza type C infections generally cause mild respiratory illness; however, types A and B are attributed to causing epidemics and their impact on health can be more severe.

Did you know? A concoction of chile pepper, honey, and tobacco was an attempt by the ancient Aztecs to treat colds. The Chinese served tea three thousand years ago to fight the cold, and today that same plant produces ephedrine, a stimulant now used to treat colds. Echinacea is one of the best-selling supplements used regularly by millions and had $300 million in sales in 2005.

Supplement it? A large meta-analysis found that taking oral vitamin C may help prevent catching a cold. Some research supports the use of elderberry extract, garlic, *Panax* ginseng, and zinc for fighting cold and flu.

Shocker Food! ─────────────────────────────

Researchers found that four gold kiwifruits daily, containing a total of about 280 mg of vitamin C, significantly reduced the severity and duration of head congestion and sore throat. Learn more about this fruit on page 43.

Apples

Apples contain many important nutrients, such as vitamin C. Dating as far back as 1947, there has been research showing that an apple a day may indeed keep the doctor away—and possible influenza, too. The pectin in apples has antiviral properties that can put a serious hurt on the influenza virus. Quercetin, a flavonoid found in the skins of apples (so leave the apple peeler in the drawer), has antiviral, anti-inflammatory, and antioxidant properties that were found to inhibit the growth of influenza virus. The total antioxidant capacity of quercetin is 3.5 times higher than that of curcumin (found in turmeric). Quercetin was also found to offset the susceptibility to infection associated with stressful exercise. Read more about apples on page 242.

Chicken Soup

Chicken soup is a good source of iron and vitamin A. It is also typically an excellent source of sodium—as much as 27 percent of the DV! Maybe Mom had good intuition all along? In the early 1200s, a Jewish scholar named Maimonides said colds should be treated with a certain "medical" brew . . . which is known today as chicken soup. The warm broth soothes a sore throat, and depending on which ingredients are added, this soup can serve as a wonderful base for other cold- and flu-fighting foods, such as carrots, which are rich in beta-carotene, and onion and garlic, which have antibacterial properties. Some research suggests that chicken soup may also work by exerting an anti-inflammatory effect on the upper respiratory tract, speeding along symptom relief and reducing the duration of the cold. An Italian study found that chicken soup had the best empirical data to support its ability to fight influenza.

Garlic

Although there's not a whole heck of a lot of other nutrients in garlic, it does contain the phytonutrients that have been found to help lower cholesterol and boost the immune system at the same time! Alliin and allicin are two sulfur compounds in garlic known for their antibiotic activity. It was Louis Pasteur who first showed how garlic juice inhibited the growth of bacteria, yeast, and fungi. A double-blind, placebo-controlled study found that those who took a garlic supplement didn't have fewer occurrences of the cold and flu, but their symptoms and duration were significantly improved. Read more about this aromatic Allium on page 160.

Elderberries

Elderberries are an excellent source of vitamin C, and a good source of vitamin A in the form of beta-carotene. These berries also contain many plant nutrients such as flavonoids, tannins, anthocyanins, and polyphenols, which help battle inflammation, cancer, and viruses. Out of all the foods and beverages featured on this list, elderberries are one of the leading foods proven for its specific benefit of stopping influenza A and B virus dead in its tracks. Much of the research done on elderberry used an extract form. In fact, a double-blind, placebo-controlled study found that symptoms from flu were relieved at average of four days earlier and that the use of medications were significantly less in those receiving elderberry extract, compared with those who received the placebo. There is even research that supports its effectiveness against H1N1, otherwise known as swine flu!

Green Tea

Green tea has long been regarded as one of the healthiest beverages you can drink, next to water. Green tea possesses antiviral properties that not only fight the influenza virus, but have also shown promise in combating herpes simplex, tobacco mosaic virus, enterovirus, rotavirus, Epstein-Barr virus, and HIV. Antifungal effects of tea have been reported against *Candida albicans* (which causes yeast infections). Page 197 has more about this remarkable beverage.

TOP 8 CANCER-FIGHTING FOODS

Featuring expert nutrition advice from Karen Collins, MS, RD, CDN, nutrition advisor for American Institute for Cancer Research

SNEAK-A-PEEK

Food	Serving	Cancer Fighting Nutrient(s)	Cancer Types Targeted
Black beans	1 cup	Fiber, anthocyanins and triterpenoids, folate, lignans, saponins	Breast, prostate, colon
Black raspberries	1 cup	Ellagitannins, ellagic acid, anthocyanins, catechins, flavonoids, vitamin C, fiber	Breast, colorectal, esophageal
Broccoli	1 cup	Glucosinolates, isothiocyanates, indoles, vitamin C, folate, beta-carotene, fiber	Lung, colorectal, stomach, breast, prostate, and other cancers
Garlic	1 clove	Allyl sulfur compounds, kaempferol, quercetin	Colorectal, stomach
Grapes	1 cup	Fiber, stilbenes, flavonoids, and resveratrol	Colon, breast, prostate, liver, lung
Spinach	1 cup	Beta-carotene, quercetin, folate, glycoglycerolipids, fiber	Esophageal, lung, colorectal, prostate
Tomatoes	1 cup	Lycopene, vitamin C, beta-carotenes, and other carotenoids	Prostate and possibly other types of cancer

Honorable mentions and best food groups: Fruit, vegetables, whole grains, fatty fish, herbs and spices

Foods that fight cancer: This list is near and dear to my heart, so you will find it a bit heftier than the others. I worked in the field of cancer care for many years and have had the honor of getting to know many experts and incredible organizations that do wonderful things. An organization that I hold in high esteem is the American Institute for Cancer Research (AICR). They support ongoing cancer research, especially in the areas of diet and lifestyle. I am honored that Karen Collins, MS, RD, CDN, their nutrition advisor, was kind enough to share her top seven foods for fighting cancer with me. Wait—eight foods are listed! Yes, that's right. I took the liberty of adding just one more food—mushrooms—because I think there is a growing amount of research supporting its role in fighting cancer.

There are many different types of cancer, so not all of them will be tackled in this list. It is also important for you to know that many other foods fight cancer and provide a similar nutrient arsenal to the ones listed here. And when I say "fight," I mean contribute to the prevention, treatment, and remission stages of cancer. But fruits and veggies can't do that battle alone. Karen shared with me that research supports that *about one-third* of our most common cancers could be prevented with a healthy diet, regular physical activity, and attaining a healthy weight. And let's not forget about the importance of proper medical care and screenings and to not do silly things, such as smoke. Avoiding harmful chemicals and toxins, getting in proper rest, and trying to avoid stress are all important items to check off your list in attempting to lower your risk for cancer. Then there is the whole genetics thing. My great-grandmother, grandmother, and mother all died from breast cancer. Is there a strong genetic connection there? You bet! But they also shared similar lifestyle choices, such as smoking, and were also overweight. What I've learned is that the choices we make in our dietary habits, and whether we decide to be physically active or not, can have a huge impact on whether cancer genes are expressed or are kept in the "off mode." Otherwise, if that wasn't the case, it would be a waste of your time and mine to share this list with you! But as you will see, many of the plant nutrients in fruits and veggies can help keep cancer genes from being expressed, within the context of an overall healthy diet and lifestyle program.

Karen also shared that AICR assembled a panel of experts who analyzed all available studies on fruits and vegetables and determined the following:

- Nonstarchy vegetables in general probably protect against cancers of the esophagus, stomach, mouth, pharynx, and larynx.
- Fruits in general probably protect against cancers of the mouth, pharynx, larynx, esophagus, stomach, and lung.

Good to know! The foods listed here provide nutrients, natural compounds, and dietary fiber that seem to act in specific ways to block or slow various stages in cancer development beyond just gene expression. Other influences, such as hormones and growth factors related to body fat and physical activity levels, also play a key role in cancer risk development. Research is increasingly showing links to cancer risk through overall eating patterns rather than specific foods or nutrients. So, it is important to keep in mind that though these foods provide a great start for a cancer battle plan, the bottom line is that they are only one part of the equation and simply adding them to your diet alone isn't an assurance that you will keep cancer at bay.

Black Beans

Cancer-fighting buddies: All dried beans, peas, and lentils can be considered together, as legumes tend to share many of the same cancer-fighting nutrients and phytochemicals. Some examples of dried beans include kidney, pinto, navy, and black beans.

Black beans contain high levels of anthocyanins and triterpenoids, powerful phytochemicals that provide amazing antioxidant power. Black beans and other legumes are among our most concentrated sources of dietary fiber, which healthful bacteria in the colon feed off to produce protective short-chain fatty acids. Dietary fiber also speeds passage of waste through the gut and dilutes the concentration of any carcinogens there. Beans are also a rich source of the B vitamin folate, which helps reduce the risk of several types of cancer due to its role in healthy cell division and ability to repair damaged cells. Lignans are under study for possible protective influences on hormones and growth factors; and saponins, which are under study for possibly reducing cancer cell growth, can bind bile acids in the gut that otherwise can promote colon cancer.

Shocker Food!

Mushrooms pack plenty of nutrients that may help protect from cancer: Arginine, beta-glucan, ergosterol (provitamin D_2), and lectin have been researched for their cancer-fighting qualities. Arginine is an amino acid associated with reduced tumor growth and increased patient survival time; beta-glucan has immunomodulatory effects and antiproliferative actions; ergosterol plays a role in making vitamin D and has many effects including inhibiting cancer cell growth; lectin can cause cell death and inhibit tumor growth. See pages 14 and 20 for more about shiitake and white mushrooms.

Studies show decreased colon cancer in animals that have been fed dried beans. Several studies link higher consumption of legumes in humans with lowered risk of colon cancer or the benign adenomas (polyps) that are the beginning of most colon cancer. In the Adventist Health Study, people consuming legumes more than two times per week were 47 percent less likely to develop colon cancer than individuals who consumed legumes less than once per week. Some research suggests that regular bean consumption may reduce the risk of prostate and breast cancer (possibly by decreasing inflammation and growth factors and increasing the self-destruction of abnormal cells). Human studies are currently inconsistent. One reason may be that most population studies in the United States include few people who eat beans frequently.

Black Raspberries

Cancer-fighting buddies: Although somewhat more studies to date suggest greater anticancer benefits of black raspberries as compared to other berries, red raspberries, strawberries, blackberries, blueberries, and cranberries all tend to share many of the same cancer-fighting nutrients and phytochemicals.

The phytochemicals ellagitannins and ellagic acid are concentrated in black raspberries and other berries, making them among the fruits with the highest levels of cancer-fighting antioxidants. Black raspberries also contain anthocyanins, catechins, and other flavonoids, as well as very high amounts of vitamin C, which protects cells' DNA by trapping free radicals and inhibiting formation of carcinogens. In a large population survey, people with a diet higher in total flavonoids and anthocyanidins (both very concentrated in berries) had lower levels of a marker of inflammation. Berries are an excellent source of dietary fiber, which reduces colon cancer risk by moving waste through the digestive tract more quickly, reducing concentration of any damaging compounds in the gut, and providing a substance that healthy gut bacteria can use to produce compounds that protect colon cells.

In laboratory studies, the phytochemicals in berries act as antioxidants to protect DNA, and they also directly interfere with cancer development at several different stages. In cell and animal studies, black raspberry and other berry extracts, and freeze-dried black raspberry powder, decrease cancer growth and stimulate self-destruction of several types of cancer cells at several stages of development. In animal studies, freeze-dried black raspberry powder reduced esophageal cancer incidence by 30 to 60 percent, and black raspberries and other berries have decreased growth of colon and mammary (breast) cancer. In a small pilot study, biopsies from people with colorectal cancer who were consuming freeze-dried black raspberry powder showed protective changes in tumor suppressor genes, as well as cancer cell growth and self-destruction. This is preliminary evidence using the equivalent of large amounts of fresh berries. See page 89 for more good news about raspberries.

Broccoli

Cancer-fighting buddies: Kale, collard, mustard greens, Brussels sprouts, rapini, broccoli sprouts (which contain up to 20 to 50 times the sulforaphane as mature broccoli), cauliflower, turnips, cabbage, and radishes.

Broccoli is probably the best known of the cruciferous vegetables, but the ones listed above will do the trick, too! All of them contain glucosinolates, which form the cancer-fighting phytonutrients isothiocyanates and indoles. These compounds can aid in decreasing inflammation, inhibit the activation and promote the detoxification of carcinogens, and decrease cancer cells' ability to spread. They also turn on tumor suppressor genes, which slow cell growth so that cell damage can be repaired, and stimulate the process called apoptosis, in which damaged cells self-destruct. Broccoli is also an excellent source of the antioxidant vitamin C, which protects cells by supporting the immune system. Additionally, broccoli is rich in phenols, a type of plant compound that decreases cell damage that could lead to cancer; and provides beta-carotene, an antioxidant that promotes cell-to-cell communication that helps control cell growth. Lastly, broccoli is rich in the B vitamin folate, which helps maintain healthy DNA and keep cancer-promoting genes "turned off."

Population studies link greater consumption of cruciferous vegetables with a lower risk of lung, colorectal, stomach, breast, prostate, and other cancers. Recent research suggests that not everyone shares equally in the benefits of the allyl sulfur compounds in broccoli due to genetic differences. However, because cruciferous vegetables supply other nutrients and fiber (see page 45), they are a smart bet for all of us to include in our meals regularly.

Garlic

Cancer-fighting buddies: Onions and leeks.

In addition to its containing the cancer-fighting flavonoids kaempferol and quercetin, crushing, chopping, or chewing garlic exposes the cloves' odorless allyl sulfur compound, alliin, to an enzyme that converts it into the active form called allicin. From allicin, a number of sulfur compounds are formed that interfere in the process of cancer development. In cell and animal studies, allyl sulfur compounds from garlic inhibited enzymes that activate carcinogens, boosted enzymes that detoxify carcinogens, enhanced DNA repair, and slowed growth and stimulated self-destruction of cancer cells without disturbing normal cells. Garlic compounds may also turn on protective genes, such as tumor suppressor genes. According to AICR's expert report, garlic probably reduces risk of colorectal cancer, and as part of the Allium vegetable family, probably lowers risk of stomach cancer. In several population studies, people who consumed more garlic were less likely to develop stomach and colorectal cancer. Other studies suggest that garlic consumption may also reduce risk of cancers of the esophagus, pancreas, breast, endometrium, and prostate, but results are mixed. The mechanisms by which garlic compounds seem to work suggest that it could help reduce risk of cancer in general, but further research is needed to understand the mechanisms.

Grapes

Cancer-fighting buddies: Cranberries, blueberries, peanuts, mulberries, bilberries, and lingonberries all contain resveratrol.

The flavonoids in the skin, flesh, and seeds of grapes protect DNA and also may inhibit cancer cells' growth and stimulate their self-destruction, as demonstrated in cell culture studies. All varieties of grapes rank high as sources of antioxidants, including the compounds stilbenes and resveratrol. Resveratrol is produced by plants to fight off fungal infections, but is a powerful antioxidant that has been shown in lab studies to thwart the growth of cancer cells. A large body of laboratory-based research that has focused on resveratrol has shown it can change cell growth signals, stimulate self-destruction of abnormal cells, and decrease their ability to spread. Resveratrol also inhibits low-grade inflammation that can set the stage for the development of colon, breast, prostate, liver, lung, and other types of cancer cells. Human studies are still very limited; however, women in two studies who consumed the most grapes or resveratrol from grapes had the least incidence of breast cancer. It is important to note that research has not supported that resveratrol from wine is protective for breast cancer. In a small pilot study, giving colon cancer patients grape powder reduced expression of a tumor-promoting gene in normal colon cells. Turn to page 288 to learn about the other nutrients in grapes.

Spinach

Cancer-fighting buddies: Beet greens and Swiss chard.

Spinach is one of many dark green leafy vegetables that contains beta-carotene and folate, but at a much higher level than even broccoli! Beta-carotene promotes cell-to-cell communication that helps control cell growth. Folate is a B vitamin that helps maintain healthy DNA and keep cancer-promoting genes "turned off." Spinach is also a rich source of vitamin C, which protects cells as an antioxidant; it also stimulates the immune system and keeps other antioxidants in their protective form. The flavonoid quercetin has been shown in cell and animal studies to slow development of several stages and types of cancer; it also boosts enzymes that detoxify carcinogens and stimulates self-destruction of cancer cells without disturbing normal cells. Glycoglycerolipids are compounds in the membranes of spinach and other green vegetable cells that contain chlorophyll. Preliminary cell and animal studies suggest these compounds may decrease cancer cells' growth and ability to spread.

Population studies that compare people with high and low amounts of beta-carotene in their diet or their blood link beta-carotene with lower risk of esophageal cancer. Studies also link foods rich in total carotenoids with lower risk of lung cancer, although research isn't completely consistent. A limited number of population studies also link higher folate consumption from food with lower pancreatic cancer risk. Many studies have linked inadequate folate intake from food with increased risk of colorectal cancer or precancerous polyps. Population studies link higher consumption of spinach with lower risk of one type of esophageal cancer and aggressive prostate cancer. Aside from its role in fighting cancer, spinach is chock-full of nutrients; see page 291.

Tomatoes

Cancer-fighting buddies: Red peppers (vitamin C), pink grapefruit, watermelon, apricots, and persimmons (carotenoids and lycopene).

Tomatoes are an example of a vegetable that might bring more to the table in its processed form than in its fresh! We often talk about "processed food" as a negative influence on nutrition because it is either removing valuable nutrients and compounds or adding unhealthy amounts of sugar or fat. When it comes to tomatoes, however, processed—meaning cooked, canned, or prepared as a juice or sauce—is good, because we can absorb the beta-carotene and lycopene much more easily from these forms. For overall health, choose low-sodium varieties. The lycopene in tomatoes is a powerful antioxidant that can prevent DNA and other cell damage. In cell studies, lycopene stimulates apoptosis (self-destruction) and decreases growth and metastasis of several types of cancer cells. Vitamin C protects cells as an antioxidant, and you will find it readily in tomato products. Tomatoes also contain beta-carotene and other carotenoids, especially the colorless compounds phytoene and phytofluene, which emerging research identifies as potentially adding protection similar to that from lycopene.

Animal studies especially link lycopene with protection from prostate cancer. Yet compared to lycopene alone, we see even lower cancer risk from whole tomato powder, which includes other carotenoids and additional compounds. Researchers are actively investigating this as a prominent example of synergy—compounds in a food acting together to produce a greater benefit than expected from adding up the effects of each individually. Of the many human studies of tomatoes and lycopene, most are observational studies of populations. Quite a few population studies and several intervention studies of prostate cancer show reduced risk or decreased PSA levels, although some large population studies do not. Some researchers suggest that inconsistencies could be reflect tomatoes' protection as most important in slowing prostate cancer from becoming a more advanced or aggressive form of the disease. See page 261 to read more about this fruit that we eat as a vegetable.

Section 3

BEST IN SHOW

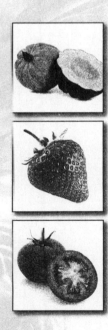

CHAPTER 9
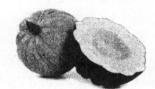
Food Category Superstars

BEST DAIRY

Food	Serving
Hard cheese	1.5 ounces
Kefir	8 ounces
Milk	8 ounces
Ricotta cheese	½ cup
Yogurt	8 ounces

Honorable mentions: Cottage cheese, sour cream, ice cream

What are the best dairy foods? Dairy is the main food group that is known for building and maintaining strong bones and reducing the risk for osteoporosis, as well as having other positive health effects. This list has the top dairy picks that are the most nutritious plus with added health benefits.

The intake of dairy products is especially important during childhood and adolescence, when bone mass is being built. Dietary recommendations found in the 2010 Dietary Guidelines for Americans support the inclusion of low- and nonfat dairy products to not only improve bone health for children and adults, but also to reduce the risk of diabetes, high blood pressure, and cardiovascular disease.

Low-fat and fat-free milk, cheese, and yogurt provide nine essential nutrients: calcium; niacin; phosphorus; potassium; protein; riboflavin; and vitamins A, D, and B$_{12}$. Diets rich in potassium may help to maintain healthy blood pressure, and dairy products, especially yogurt, fluid milk, and soy milk, provide potassium. Vitamin D functions in the body to maintain proper levels of calcium and phosphorous, thereby helping to build and maintain bones. Vitamin D–fortified milks and soy milks are good sources of this nutrient; other sources, when vitamin D–fortified, include yogurt and ready-to-eat breakfast cereals.

When comparing different cow's milk—whole vs. 2% vs. skim, and so on—there is no difference in calcium, vitamin D, and other nutrients. These are not skimmed away with the fat; the only difference is that you're giving your body more calories and unhealthy fat when you choose whole over 2% milk.

HOW MUCH IS ENOUGH?

You may be familiar with the slogan "3-a-day." Dairy products are the primary source of calcium in the American diet, and consuming three cups or the equivalent of dairy products per day, if you are aged nine or older, can help meet your daily calcium needs. Those three low- or nonfat dairy servings have also been found to play a role in maintaining a healthy weight and promote healthy blood pressure control, among other health benefits!

Daily Recommendation for Milk					
Age (years)	Children (cups/day)	Males (cups/day)	Females (cups/day)	Pregnancy (cups/day)	Lactation (cups/day)
2–3	2				
4–8	2½				
9–13		3	3		
14–18		3	3	3	3
19–30		3	3	3	3
31–50		3	3	3	3
51+ years		3	3		

SOURCE: MyPlate.gov

Did you know? Domestication of a wild relative of today's cow, known as an aurochs, is thought to have begun back in 8000 to 6000 BC in the Fertile Crescent. But it wasn't until 1624 that the first cows arrived in America, in Plymouth, Massachusetts.

Shocker Food! ———

Flavored milk is often targeted as a contributor toward childhood obesity, though research to date does not support this premise. In fact, studies show that:

- Kids drink more milk when it's flavored.
- No nutrients are lost when flavoring is added to white milk—it still contains all of the nine essential nutrients that milk is known for!
- Drinking low-fat or fat-free flavored milk helps fill the nutrient void that kids are experiencing today—namely, not getting enough of calcium, potassium, and magnesium as well as vitamin D.
- Lastly, research shows that kids who drink flavored milk meet more of their nutritional needs without consuming more added sugar, fat, or calories than non-milk drinkers. And kids who drink flavored milk are *not* heavier than those kids who don't! Besides, low-fat chocolate milk is the most popular milk choice in schools—not offering it only limits kids' choices for healthy beverages.

Low-fat chocolate milk may be a preferred beverage among athletes, too, as studies are showing that drinking chocolate milk between exercise sessions improves recovery and enables athletes to perform longer until they became fatigued. Low-fat chocolate milk is an excellent source of calcium, phosphorus, and riboflavin, and a good source of vitamins A and D.

Hard Cheese

If you are looking for the most calcium in the smallest package, cheese is your best bet. And not all cheese is created equal in the calcium department. Hard cheeses contain the most calcium, followed by semihard, soft, then fresh. The calcium in cheese helps relieve PMS symptoms, which is really good news! A Finnish study found that cheese-eating adolescent girls had stronger bones compared to than those who did not. Some hard cheese varieties, such as Parmigiano-Reggiano, are not only rich in pro-tein and calcium but also possess prebiotic and probiotic properties; and one and a half ounces of aged Parmesan cheese is an excellent source of calcium (500 mg!), phosphorus, and protein. See pages 61 and 62 for more about hard cheese and Parmesan cheese.

> It takes ten pounds of cow's milk to make one pound of cheese!

Kefir

If you haven't tried it before, kefir is a kind of a cross between yogurt and milk, with a pleasant creamy consistency and a sweet, tangy taste. There are friendly bacteria that form naturally when kefir is made that help promote healthy digestion. Kefiran, a plant nutrient that is the sub-ject of much research, is produced by the bacteria Lactobacillus kefira-nofaciens, found in kefir grains. See page 289 for the rich roster of nutrients in kefir. In addition to its digestive benefits, kefir also has been found to help bone health by providing 25 percent of the RDA for vita-min D and 30 percent for calcium. A recent study also found potential cancer-slowing power with drinking kefir. The *Journal of Cancer Man-agement and Research* featured a study in which researchers found that kefir inhibited proliferation of specific cancer cells. Kefir is also thought to enhance immune function, reduce inflammation, and lower blood pressure and cholesterol.

Milk

Milk does a body good and apparently in more ways than just protecting our bone structure. In a meta-analysis of nineteen different studies that looked at milk and dairy consumption and its relationship to colon cancer risk, those men and women who consumed the higher end of dairy (three or more servings per day) had the lowest risk for colon cancer. Turn to page 289 for more about the many benefits of milk.

Ricotta Cheese

The whey protein in ricotta cheese has been demonstrated to be beneficial in lowering high blood pressure that could lead to stroke. Fermented whey proteins have been found to reduce the harmful bacteria *H. pylori,* which may benefit digestive health. An animal study found that the whey proteins in cheese helped reduce inflammation associated with colitis. Also, whey is a valuable protein for increasing lean muscle mass. Learn more about ricotta on page 94.

Yogurt

Of all dairy products, yogurt is most concentrated in both potassium and calcium. The combination of these two minerals is particularly beneficial in preventing bone loss. Relatively new to the yogurt scene, Greek yogurt is another great option for getting a serving of dairy. Low-fat Greek yogurt is an excellent source of calcium (up to 30 percent of the DV), phosphorus, protein (upward of 23 g per cup!), riboflavin (up to 30 percent of the DV), vitamin B_{12}, and zinc. It is a good source of magnesium, pantothenic acid, and potassium. See page 13 for more about yogurt. Besides its amazing nutrition profile, yogurt has some incredible health benefits, too. Making yogurt part of a regular diet has been shown to enhance immune function, promote healthy digestion, and improve oral health. In addition, studies have shown that eating a low-fat variety of dairy products lowers the incidence of type 2 diabetes. A study of 82,076 postmenopausal women found that those who consumed low-fat dairy products had a much lower risk of developing type 2 diabetes, especially if those women were obese. Even more amazing was that there was even a stronger association for those women who ate yogurt with reducing the risk for diabetes!

BEST GRAINS

SNEAK-A-PEEK

Food (Cooked)	Serving
Amaranth	½ cup
Barley	½ cup
Oats	½ cup
Quinoa	½ cup
Teff	½ cup
Triticale	½ cup
Wheat	½ cup

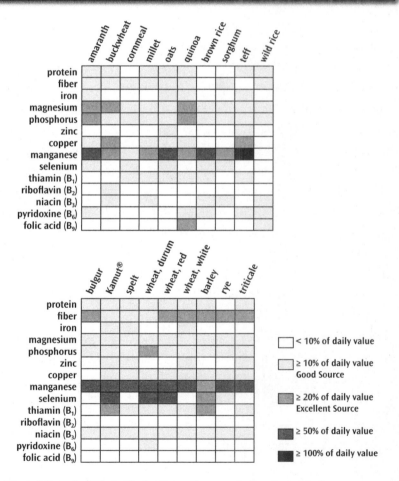

SOURCE: Adapted from the Whole Grains Council, www.wholegrainscouncil.org.

Honorable mentions: Buckwheat, millet, rye, brown rice, wild rice, sorghum, corn

Worth mentioning: In determining the best grains for you, consider more than just nutrient density. For example, if these grains were ranked strictly by nutrient content alone, barley would have ranked number two and oats number seven. However, when you factor in evidence-based health benefits, barley and oats would be neck and neck for the lead! The overarching theme here is to choose a variety of whole grains in your diet, as each brings something different and healthy to the table—they're all great!

What are whole grains and why are they good for you? According to the Whole Grains Council, the definition of *whole grain* is fairly straightforward: " . . . 100% of the original kernel—all of the bran, germ, and endosperm— must be present to qualify as a whole grain."

Health experts used to hang their hat on the fiber content of whole grains as the payoff, but research shows the health benefits of eating whole grains go well beyond the fiber content. The unique nutrient package, including their macro-, micro-, and phytonutrients, contribute to whole grains' overall health benefits. A recent meta-analysis found that whole grains play an important role in lowering the risk of chronic diseases, such as coronary heart disease, diabetes, and cancer, and also contribute to body weight management and gastrointestinal health. Studies show that swapping in whole grains to replace refined grains lowers the risk of many chronic diseases. While benefits are most pronounced for those consuming at least three servings daily, some studies show reduced risks from as little as one serving daily. Researchers at Tufts University conducted a study involving nearly three thousand men and women and found that adults who ate three or more serving of whole grains and limited refined grain items to one daily serving or less had 10 percent less belly fat than those who didn't eat this way. Unfortunately, according to a 2010 study in the *Journal of the American Dietetic Association*, only one in twenty adults are consuming enough whole grains. That's really going against the grain!

HOW MUCH IS ENOUGH?

According to the USDA MyPlate guidelines, the amount of whole grains that you need to derive health benefits depends on your age, sex, and level of physical activity. In general, it is suggested to make at least half of your grain intake whole. Below, each ounce is equivalent to ½ cup of cooked grain.

Daily Recommendation for Grains			
Age (years)	Children (ounces)	Males (ounces)	Females (ounces)
2–3	3 1½*		
4–8	5 2½*		
9–13		6 3*	5 3*
14–18		8 4*	6 3*
19–30		8 4*	6 3*
31–50		7 3½*	6 3*
51+		6 3*	5 3*

*Minimum daily amount. Adapted from www.choosemyplate.gov; these amounts are appropriate for individuals who get less than thirty minutes per day of moderate physical activity, beyond normal daily activities. Those who are more physically active may be able to consume more while staying within calorie needs.

Did you know? Canary seed, Job's tears, montina, timothy, and fonio are considered whole grains but were not included in this review, as they are not as commonly consumed. Oil seeds and legumes such as flax, chia, sunflower, soy, chickpeas, and so on are not considered whole grains by the Whole Grain Council nor the USDA or the FDA, despite their sometimes being used as grains, such as in the form of flours. Also, amaranth, quinoa, and buckwheat are considered "pseudo-grains"; because they are commonly sold as cereal grains and their nutritional profile and preparation are similar to those of grains, they were included in the review.

Amaranth

Amaranth is a good source of protein, and like quinoa, contains greater amounts of amino acids than other grains. Amaranth is an excellent source of magnesium, manganese, and phosphorus, and a good source of copper, fiber, iron, and vitamin B_6. It has more nutrients—such as fiber, iron, and magnesium—than other gluten-free grains. Amaranth is a rich source of tannins and phytosterols, which may help combat a variety of cancers and heart disease. It is also rich in lunasin, a peptide that has anti-cancer properties.

Barley

See page 183 for the full profile on barley. Its beta-glucans reduce cholesterol, help control blood sugar, and improve immune system function; and some recent research suggests that those same beta-glucans may help protect the body against collateral damage to healthy cells caused by the ravages of chemotherapy, radiation therapy, and nuclear exposure. Other well-researched benefits of barley include reducing blood pressure, lowering LDL cholesterol, possibly lessening the risk of heart disease, helping control blood glucose, promoting satiety, and reducing belly fat.

> The English are indebted to the barley grain for their measurement system. King Edward II placed three grains of barley end to end and exclaimed that the total measurement would be equivalent to an inch. All other English distance measures were based on this.

Oats

Whether steel cut, old-fashioned rolled, or instant, all forms of oats contain the three components that make a whole grain. Read more about their nutritional benefits on page 160. Oats also contain polyphenols called avenanthramides, which are antioxidants that reduce inflammation and soothe itching—which is why oat baths are recommended for the latter condition. No other grain has been researched more than oats for its cholesterol-lowering abilities. Besides the ability to lower total and LDL cholesterol, thus reducing the risk of heart disease, oats also show promise for satiety and weight control, lowering blood pressure, blood glucose management, and promoting regularity due to their fiber content.

Quinoa

Botanically, quinoa is a relative of Swiss chard and beets, and technically is not a true whole grain. Aside from its many other nutrients (see page 290), it is one of the only plant foods that is a complete protein, because it contains all the essential amino acids. Quinoa is relatively new when it comes to research, but benefits shown thus far include reducing the risk for diabetes and contributing to satiety. Quinoa also contains the highest level of potassium of all the whole grains, which aids blood pressure.

Teff

Thanks to its small size, you will never have to worry about teff's being stripped of its outside bran layer, because it is simply too small to mill. Teff is largely unknown outside of Ethiopia, India, and Australia but is becoming more and more popular because of its versatility and nutrition and health benefits, including blood glucose management, weight control, and colon health. Turn to page 292 for a profile of its nutrients.

Triticale

Triticale is a fairly new hybrid of wheat and rye that was first developed over one hundred years ago in Scotland to grow in more challenging climates. The first attempt produced a sterile grain, but then a German botanist perfected the hybridization process. After experiencing a burst of popularity in the 1970s, triticale hasn't really caught on, though. Because it requires little help from pesticides and reduces soil erosion, this grain lends itself well to organic farming. Triticale is an excellent source of fiber and manganese, and a good source of copper, magnesium, niacin, phosphorus, protein, thiamine, and zinc. Triticale has similar health benefits to rye, such as improving regularity and satiety, and weight and blood sugar management. Recently, the bran of triticale was found to possess strong prebiotic properties (helps stimulate the growth of friendly bacteria) and also this grain ranks high on the ORAC scale, a system that determines antioxidant activity.

Wheat

This would qualify as a shocker food, as it seems many of the nation's health woes have been pinned lately on this whole-grain staple. Truth is, if you don't have an allergy or intolerance to it, whole wheat is one of the healthiest grains on earth and is responsible for providing significant nutrition to millions of people around the globe every day. Wheat, encompassing such grains as durum, kamut, and spelt, is by far the most common grain used in breads, pastas, and other grain foods eaten in the United States. Whole wheat is an excellent source of fiber, manganese, phosphorus, and selenium, and a good source of copper, magnesium, niacin, protein, thiamine, and vitamin B_6. Most of the studies espousing the benefits of whole grains include whole wheat as the focal grain. Benefits of including whole wheat in the diet include reducing the risk of heart disease by 25 to 28 percent, lowering the risk of stroke by 30 to 36 percent, lessening the risk of type 2 diabetes by 21 to 30 percent, weight maintenance, reducing the risk of asthma, promoting blood pressure levels, and lessening the risk of inflammatory disease.

BEST GLUTEN-FREE GRAINS

SNEAK-A-PEEK

Food (Cooked)	Serving
Amaranth	½ cup
Buckwheat	½ cup
Millet	½ cup
Oats	½ cup
Quinoa	½ cup
Sorghum	½ cup
Teff	½ cup

Honorable mentions: Montina, wild rice

What is gluten and why eat gluten-free? Over 21 million people follow a gluten-free diet. While many of those who follow this diet have been diagnosed with celiac disease or gluten sensitivity, many others believe it is simply a healthier way to eat, though evidence-based research is lacking to support this assumption.

For the over 3 million who have been diagnosed with celiac disease, gluten-free eating is an absolute necessity. Celiac disease is a genetically based autoimmune disorder characterized by an immune response to gluten, a protein found in grains such as barley, rye, and wheat and its relatives, such as triticale, spelt, kamut, and faro. Durum, bulgur, couscous, and semolina are also wheat, and therefore contain gluten. Ingested gluten causes damage by generating an allergic inflammatory reaction in the small intestine. Growing need and interest has created a booming market for gluten-free foods and in 2010, gluten-free product sales accounted for $2.64 billion in sales.

Did you know? According to Alesso Fassano, MD, director of the University of Maryland Center for Celiac Research, an estimated 1 in 133 Americans have celiac disease and up to 95 percent of them don't even know they have it.

Amaranth

This grain has a sweet, nutty flavor and lends a slight crunch to a dish. It can be bought as flour or seeds. See page 285 to learn about amaranth's nutritional benefits. In addition, it contains squalene, an antioxidant that may prevent cancer growth and counteract high cholesterol. This powerful grain may also help control high blood sugar.

Buckwheat

Buckwheat is actually a fruit! It is a seed related to the rhubarb plant, and bees make honey from its flowers. Its groats are commonly used in western Asia and Eastern Europe. Buckwheat is an excellent source of choline and a good source of magnesium. It also contains B vitamins, fiber, magnesium, manganese, selenium, vitamin E, and zinc, and is plentiful in the phyto-nutrients lignans, phenolic acids, phytic acid, and rutin. A review study found that experiments in both animals and humans demonstrated that buckwheat flour may help with fighting, controlling, or improving diabetes, obesity, hypertension, hypercholesterolemia, and constipation.

Millet

Millet is a tiny yellow grain with a mild, sweet flavor. It is a good source of choline and contains many nutrients, including copper, magnesium, manganese, phosphorus, and zinc. Millet also contains the carotenoids lutein and zeaxanthin, which are essential for normal vision and have been found to protect against macular degeneration. Millet, like many other whole grains, may help control cholesterol and blood sugar levels.

Oats

Many who follow a gluten-free diet are often told that oats contain gluten. The truth is they are and always have been gluten free. The trouble with oats is guilt by association. Some oat products on the market may have been cross-contaminated with gluten-containing grains at the point of manufacturing, or during transport by being trucked in containers that once contained gluten-containing grains. Solution? Look for brands that are certified gluten free!

Read up on the excellent health profile of this popular grain.

Quinoa

Because of its protein and fiber content, one of the perks of eating quinoa is satiety. Quinoa has many different variations of saponins, which are phytochemicals found to have anticancer and anti-inflammatory properties and inhibit cholesterol absorption. Turn to page 230 for more about this newly popular grain.

Quinoa was a staple food in ancient civilizations and cultivated in the South American Andes since at least 3000 BC.

Sorghum

There are many varieties of sorghum, but the one we use like a grain is technically considered a grass. Although a staple for human consumption in Africa, sorghum is commonly used for animal food; only recently has it come into favor in the West as a great grain alternative for the gluten challenged. A cell study found that sorghum contains a variety of flavonoids and proanthocyanidins that inhibit the action of aromatase, which is a key enzyme that helps with the production of estrogen. Aromatase inhibitors are commonly used in the treatment of estrogen-driven breast cancer.

Teff

Tiny teff is an excellent source of many nutrients (see page 292). Apart from use in its native Africa, teff is a popular gluten-free grain in the Netherlands. In a survey of nearly eight thousand members of the Dutch Celiac Disease Society, teff was reported to be a favorite because celiac sufferers experience a significant reduction in symptoms and stated that they simply felt better.

BEST NUTS

SNEAK-A-PEEK

Food	Serving
Almonds	1 ounce
Brazil nuts	1 ounce
Hazelnuts	1 ounce
Peanuts	1 ounce
Pecans	1 ounce
Pistachios	1 ounce
Walnuts	1 ounce

Honorable mentions: Macadamias, chestnuts, cashews

What are nuts and why should you eat them? Technically, nuts grow on trees; soy nuts and peanuts are legumes. But for the purposes of this list, peanuts will be included because they are high in fat and are thought of as nuts by consumers.

Nuts are quite nutritious, featuring an array of vitamins and minerals, plus they contain varying amounts of special plant nutrients that work as antioxidants, reduce inflammation, fight cancer and keep cancer cells from multiplying, help lower cholesterol, and combat heart disease. These plant chemicals include alkylphenols, carotenoids, flavonoids, lignans, phenolic acids, phytates, phytosterols, proanthocyanidins, sphingolipids, and stilbenes. The good news is that very little of nuts' nutrition are compromised during the roasting process. Nuts also contain heart-healthy fats as their main source of calories, while low in saturated fat and without any trans fats whatsoever. Research suggests that those populations that consume nuts regularly and in moderation do a better job of achieving and maintaining a healthy weight than do those who are not regular nut eaters. Guess that busts the age-old fattening myth that surrounds nuts! Another plus: Nuts contain protein and fiber, which help keep you full and satisfied.

Did you know? Scientific evidence suggests, but does not prove, that eating 1.5 ounces per day of most nuts, as part of a diet low in saturated fat and cholesterol, may reduce the risk of heart disease.

Shocker Food!

Pine nuts are also included under the qualified heart health claim for nuts. Although low in fiber, they are one of the richest sources of manganese and polyunsaturated fats. For a fuller profile of this little gem, see page 87. It bears repeating to be careful when eating them, as pine nuts have been found to be more allergenic than most nuts.

Almonds

You get twenty-three kernels (a handful) in a 1-ounce serving of almonds and they clock in at 160 calories per serving. In addition to being supernutritious (see page 285), they also are rich in heart-healthy monounsaturated

Almonds are believed to have originated in China and Central Asia. The nut comes from a flowering tree that is pollinated by bees. What is unique about almonds is that the nut itself lies within the fruit that grows on the tree. The young green raw almond is a prized nut and is sold during a limited season.

fats and contain plant nutrients such as flavanols, phytosterols, and proanthocyanins. Nine clinical studies support that almonds can help maintain healthy cholesterol levels as part of a diet low in saturated fat. Additional research has demonstrated that almonds possess prebiotic properties that help bolster a healthy digestive tract as well as supporting proper immune function. Almond research has also shown benefits in areas of health including polycystic ovary syndrome (PCOS), diabetes, high blood pressure, weight management, digestion, and antimicrobial (bacteria-killing) abilities.

Brazil Nuts

Brazil nuts are packed with nutrients (see page 286) but also calories—a 1-ounce serving (6 kernels) will set you back 190 calories. Brazil nuts are absolutely brimming with the mineral selenium, the highest of any nut! One ounce has over 700 percent of the daily recommendation! Research has found that daily consumption can effectively increase selenium status—one study saw an improvement with just two nuts a day!

Brazil nuts grow in clusters inside a pod that looks like a coconut, on trees in the Amazon rainforest. These nuts first came into notoriety in 1569, when Spanish troops feasted on the delicious nuts to regain their strength.

Hazelnuts

A 1-ounce serving of hazelnuts (about twenty-one whole kernels, which roll in at 180 calories) is high in vitamins and minerals (see page 288), particularly folate, which isn't true of all nuts. Folate is a key nutrient during pregnancy and also helps prevent anemia. A study demonstrated that just a small serving of hazelnuts daily can have a significant cholesterol-lowering effect. Besides, hazelnuts are high in heart-healthy monounsaturated fat, and have the highest proanthocyanidin content of any tree nut—a powerful anti-inflammatory that helps protect the heart. These compounds are also known for helping to reduce the risk of blood clotting and urinary tract infections.

Filbert is the correct name for this nut, derived from the name of a French saint, Philibert. *Hazelnut*, the more popular name, was coined by the English, and in 1981, the Oregon Filbert Commission decided to conform to the common standard and began using the term *hazelnut*.

Peanuts

As opposed to tree nuts, peanuts grow underground. A 1-ounce serving of peanuts provides 170 calories and a wealth of nutrients (see page 289). They are rich in the amino acid arginine, which helps expand blood vessels and decrease blood pressure. Peanuts contain high levels of phytosterols that block cholesterol from being absorbed into the bloodstream and may also have cancer-preventative properties. In a study of Seventh-Day Adventists, regular peanut consumption was inversely associated with death from ischemic heart disease. And if you don't want to turn to a glass of wine to get a dose of heart-healthy resveratrol, a study published in the *Journal of Agricultural and Food Chemistry* found that peanuts contain amounts that rival what's in red wine. Extensive research also shows other health benefits of eating peanuts, including but not limited to combating diabetes, cancer, inflammation, and high blood pressure.

The peanut plant is thought to have come from South America and migrated to distant lands via European explorers. Although peanuts were grown in the southern regions of North America from the time of colonialists, significant production of peanuts didn't occur in the United States until the early 1900s, when Dr. George Washington Carver discovered over three hundred uses for the legume! Peanut butter and a variety of other peanut-based products, including a need for more plant oils during World War I, helped bring attention to the industry.

Pecans

There are over one thousand different kinds of pecans, varying in taste and size, but all are nutritious and contain more than nineteen vitamins and minerals (see page 115). A 1-ounce serving (about 19 halves) contains 200 calories. Naturally occurring antioxidants in pecans may help contribute to heart health and disease prevention, according to a study at Loma Linda University. A research project found that the vitamin E levels of study participants whose meals included pecans doubled in the eight hours after dining, their antioxidant levels also increased after the meals, and their oxidized LDL cholesterol decreased by up to 33 percent during that same period. More research from Loma Linda University found that adding just a handful of pecans to the diet each day may help keep oxidized LDL cholesterol associated with coronary heart disease at bay. Additional research demonstrates pecans' ability to help manage weight, increase metabolic rates, and enhance satiety.

> Pecans can be traced back to the sixteenth century. They are the only tree nut native to North America. *Pecan* is a Native American word meaning "all nuts requiring a stone to crack."

Pistachios

A 1-ounce serving of pistachios (49 kernels) provides 170 calories and a variety of vitamins and minerals (see page 136). Almost 90 percent of the fat found in pistachios is the healthy mono- and polyunsaturated fat. Research supports pistachios' ability to improve lipid profiles that affect the heart, promote antioxidant and anti-inflammatory activity, stabilize glycemic control, protect endothelial function, and control body weight, when consumed in moderation.

> Pistachios grow in heavy, grapelike clusters, and when they ripen, the kernel fills the inside of the shell so quickly that it splits the shell. In America, imported pistachios were once dyed red to disguise shell imperfections and make the nuts stand out in vending machines.

Walnuts

Walnuts are unique compared to other nuts because they are composed predominantly of polyunsaturated fatty acids, including the omega-3 fat alpha linolenic acid, rather than monounsaturated fatty acids. A 1-ounce serving of walnuts (about 14 halves) contains 190 calories. In addition to supplying a wealth of minerals (see page 119), two recent studies found that walnuts contained more antioxidants than any other nut as well as, overall, coming in second place only to blackberries, out of 1,113 different foods. Walnuts also contain the "sleep hormone" melatonin (see page 280). Nearly two decades of research conducted worldwide have shown that walnuts may benefit heart health, diabetes, cancer, cognition, aging, and metabolic syndrome. A recent study published in the *American Journal of Clinical Nutrition* found that walnuts rivaled fatty fish for their ability to lower specific blood markers associated with coronary heart disease. The study found that a diet including walnuts was more powerful in reducing total and LDL cholesterol when compared to fatty fish.

BEST FRUITS

SNEAK-A-PEEK

Food	Serving
Apples	1 small
Apricots	4 small
Bananas	1 cup
Blueberries	1 cup
Cherries	1 cup
Cranberries (fresh) Cranberries (dried)	1 cup ½ cup
Elderberries	1 cup
Figs (fresh) Figs (dried)	1 cup ½ cup
Grapes Raisins	1 cup ½ cup

continues

continued

Food	Serving
Guavas	1 cup
Kiwis	1 cup
Oranges Orange juice	1 large 1 cup
Papayas	1 cup
Pears	1 medium
Pineapples	1 cup
Plums (fresh) Prunes	1 cup ¼ cup
Raspberries	1 cup
Sapodillas	1 cup
Strawberries	1 cup
Watermelon	1 cup

Honorable mentions: All others! There's no such thing as a bad fruit!

What are fruits and why should you eat them? You may be hoping that I can settle the argument once and for all of what constitutes a fruit—is avocado or tomato a fruit or a vegetable?

Well, the classification of fruits falls into two general areas: fleshy and dry fruits. Fleshy fruits are often sweet and juicy and consist of living cells, though avocado and olives, which are not sweet (the answer to your first question), are an exception to this rule. Dry fruits consist of two subcategories: dehiscent (dead cells that split open at maturity, such as legumes) and indehiscent fruit (dead cells that don't split open—nuts, for example; however cashews are seeds, not fruits). Then there is another level of sophistication: whether the fruit comes from lower part of the plant called the ovary, or from other parts of the plant. Those that come from another part of the plant are often referred to as "false fruits." The strawberry is a good example of this: the part that people enjoy, which is the red fleshy part, is just a receptacle—the two hundred–odd seedlike thingys that stud the flesh, and which are called achenes, are actually the fruit. Freaky but good! For this list, we will consider only fleshy fruits and berries.

Unfortunately, it is estimated that fewer than 6 percent of the U.S. population are following all of the dietary guidelines, which include strong encouragement to make half of our plate fruits and vegetables. Such recommendations are based in science and not just intuition, as those populations that consume the most produce have lower rates of heart disease, cancer, diabetes, obesity, and the list goes on. Fruits contain many essential vitamins, minerals, and other nutrients that combat disease, but also offer phytochemicals that may be doing the bulk of the disease fighting.

It's a good idea not to follow a "unifruit" diet, such as the once-popular grapefruit diet. Variety is the spice of life . . . and a good and healthy life, at that! The greater the diversity, the more likely your body will enjoy not only all the unique flavors that fruit has to offer but also their variety of health benefits, such as reduced risk of heart attack and stroke, certain types of cancers, obesity, type 2 diabetes, high blood pressure, the development of kidney stones, and bone loss.

HOW MUCH IS ENOUGH?

According to the USDA MyPlate recommendations, fruit requirements are dependent on your level of physical activity, age, and gender:

Daily Recommendation for Fruit			
Age (years)	Children (cups/day)	Males (cups/day)	Females (cups/day)
2–3	1		
4–8	1–1½		
9–13		1½	1½
14–18		2	1½
19–30		2	2
31–50		2	1½
51+		2	1½

These amounts are appropriate for individuals who get less than thirty minutes per day of moderate physical activity, beyond normal daily activities. Those who are more physically active may be able to consume more while staying within calorie needs.

Did you know? Most fruits are naturally low in fat, sodium, and calories. None have cholesterol. Fruits are sources of many essential nutrients that are underconsumed, including fiber, folate, potassium, and vitamin C.

Apples

According to the USDA, the nutritional content will vary slightly depending on their variety and size. Don't peel your apple—two-thirds of the fiber and lots of antioxidants are found in the peel. Antioxidants help reduce damage to cells, which can trigger some diseases. Apples' pectin, a soluble fiber, helps prevent cholesterol buildup in the lining of blood vessel walls, thus reducing the incidence of atherosclerosis and heart disease; while their insoluble fiber provides bulk in the intestinal tract, holding water to cleanse and move food quickly through the digestive system. A 2008 study by Victor Fulgoni, PhD, found that adults who eat apples and apple products have smaller waistlines that indicate less abdominal fat, lower blood pressure, and a reduced risk for developing metabolic syndrome.

> The crab apple is the only apple that is native to North America, but you can find a total of over 2,500 different kinds of apples growing in all fifty states! Worldwide, there are over 7,500 varieties of apples.

Apricots

The beta-carotene content of apricots can vary greatly depending on the cultivar, mainly related to color. The darker red/orange-colored varieties have been found to contain up to 16,500 mcg of beta-carotene per 100 grams of fruit! Aside from its other nutrients (see page 285), apricots also contain ten different polyphenols, each possessing significant antioxidant properties: caffeic acid, chlorogenic acid, ferulic acid, gallic acid, p-aminobenzoic acid, p-coumaric acid, procatechinic acid, quercetin, rutin, and vanillin. These polyphenols may help fight cancer and heart disease, and even build bones.

> Ever wonder why apricots are so aromatic? Like apples, cherries, peaches, pears, plums, raspberries, and strawberries, they belong to the Rosaceae family—the same family as roses.

Bananas

The biggest herb in the world produces one of the most popular fruits in America. Bananas are an excellent source of vitamins and minerals (see page 286), especially potassium. Many are unaware that bananas and the skin they come in have amazing antifungal and antibiotic properties that act against bad *Mycobacteria*. Feel-good chemicals called neurotransmitters that occur in the brain can also be found in bananas: dopamine, norepinephrine, and serotonin are present in the ripe peel and also the fruit itself. Even green bananas come to the table bearing health benefits. When they are green, bananas are an excellent source of resistant starch (which gets its name from passing through the small intestine undigested), which helps control blood glucose and lower cholesterol, and may play a role in fighting colon cancer.

> Did you know rubbing banana peel on your skin helps repel mosquitoes?

Blueberries

At only 80 calories per cup, blueberries are an excellent source of vitamins, minerals, and fiber (see page 286). Researcher Ronald Prior, PhD, found that a 1-cup serving of wild blueberries had more total antioxidant capacity than any other berry or other types of fruit. Blueberries may help prevent and reverse age-related cognitive decline, including Alzheimer's, as was discovered in animal research. It has been found in human research that blueberries help maintain memory function and improve mood in older adults with early memory decline.

Cherries

Cherries contain a host of nutrients (see page 287), including cancer-fighting amygdalin; pain-relieving anthocyanins; boron, which builds strong bones; and quercetin, which also helps with bone building and maintains heart health. A good chunk of scientific literature supports cherries' role in helping to relieve painful inflammatory conditions, such as postexercise muscle pain, heart disease, and gouty arthritis. It is believed that the anthocyanins that give cherries their bright red color are responsible for extinguishing the flames of inflammation but not of desire. In fact, cherries may help stimulate nitric oxide production in arteries, allowing more blood flow to all the right places.

Cranberries

Turn to page 192 for the many benefits of cranberries. Research has demonstrated regular cranberry consumption supports urinary tract and heart health. Not only can cranberries do a smack-down on *E. coli* bacteria associated with urinary tract infections, but studies have found that cranberry also destroys *H. pylori* bacteria, a major contributor to ulcers and a risk for stomach cancer.

Elderberries

Elderberries are loaded with nutrients (see page 209) and worth seeking out. Although not often available fresh in stores, you can find them in jams and jellies, and also in extract form in your local health food store. In addition to elderberries' fighting a variety of strains of influenza, cell studies indicate that this fruit contains lectins that may help ward off gallbladder cancer. A Canadian animal study found that when fish oil and elderberries were combined and fed to hamsters, the lipid-lowering effects were much greater than from just fish oil alone.

Figs

Dried figs are a dense source of heart healthy polyphenols and an excellent source of numerous vitamins and minerals (see page 133). Research studies have found that dried figs had substantially higher content of disease-fighting and anti-inflammatory phenolic compounds than did their fresh counterpart.

Grapes and Raisins

Fresh red or green grapes are a good source of vitamins B$_6$ and K; their resveratrol, a polyphenol, has antioxidant and anticancer properties. Raisins are an excellent source of iron and a good source of fiber, phosphorus, and potassium. And grape juice is also nutritious (see page 288). Many cell and animal studies have found grapes contribute to the health of the brain, eyes, bladder, and liver, and also support immune health, while helping protect against cervical and breast cancer. Specific to Concord grapes and grape juice, research has discovered that adding grape juice to the diet supports cardiovascular health by helping by slowing down the oxidation rate of LDL cholesterol and keeping arteries flexible. Healthy arteries also means good news for regulating blood pressure—two human studies have shown significant reductions in blood pressure in hypertensive subjects that consume grape juice. Specific to raisins, human research supports improved heart health; reduced inflammation markers; and lowered total and LDL cholesterol, C-reactive protein, and blood pressure. Many oral health experts recommend avoiding such foods as raisins because they feel their stickiness may contribute to the promotion of cavity formation. However, a study out of the University of Illinois College of Dentistry found that raisins are rich in the phytochemical oleanolic acid, which shows no mercy in its killing ability of cavity and plaque-promoting bacteria such as *Streptococcus mutans*.

Guavas

All hail the king of vitamin C! Aside from this and other vitamins and minerals (see page 288), guavas contain a vast amount of phytonutrients, such as essential oils, flavonoids, lectins, phenols, saponins, tannins, and triterpenes. Recent animal research supports a role of guava fruit and its leaves, which are rich in flavonoids and phenolic acids, in protecting kidney health against the negative effects of diabetes. Mice fed guava had significantly reduced blood urea nitrogen (BUN), a marker of kidney damage, compared to those that weren't fed guava.

Kiwis

Among its many nutrients (see page 43), kiwifruits contain lutein, which is beneficial in eye health maintenance and may reduce the risk of night blindness and macular degeneration. A Japanese study found that kiwi fruit had stronger antioxidant effects than oranges and grapefruit and that the gold variety of kiwi had stronger antioxidant effects than green kiwifruit. Kiwifruit may block early lipid oxidation that leads to hardening of the arteries. They are also an irritable bowel sufferer's best friend (see page 44).

Oranges and Orange Juice

A large, sweet orange is an excellent source of vitamin C, and a good source of fiber, folate, and thiamine. Read about the many benefits of orange juice on pages 44, 165, and 181. Although it sometimes gets a bad rap as being a "smoking gun" in contributing to childhood obesity, in a study that looked at the consumption of 100 percent orange juice in 7,250 children ranging from two to eighteen years of age, among those kids who drank orange juice, the usual intake averaged only about 10 ounces a day. Even though calorie consumption was higher than those kids who didn't drink orange juice regularly, there were no differences in weight, BMI, or risk of being overweight or obese between kids who drank orange juice and those who didn't. Kids who drank orange juice also had higher intakes of such nutrients as folate, magnesium, and vitamins A and C. The consumers also had higher intakes of total fruit, fruit juice, and whole fruit.

Oranges belong to the genus *Citrus,* of the family Rutaceae. There are several varieties, such as sweet orange (*C. sinensis*); the Seville, or bitter, orange (*C. aurantium*); the bergamot orange (*C. bergamia*); and mandarin orange (*C. reticulate*), of which clementines and tangerines are subspecies.

Papayas

Nutritious papayas (see page 289) are rich in the protein-digestive enzymes papain and chymopapain. In a human cell study, papaya was found to increase the effectiveness of immune soldiers called T cells, in combating inflammation. This

> Papayas belong to the berry family and are believed to be native to southern Mexico and Central America.

may have to do with the high levels of anti-inflammatory enzymes and nutrients naturally found in papaya. PS: The black seeds that we usually throw away are edible and have a spicy peppery taste!

Pears

Read pears' nutritional profile on page 289. In a study of 411 overweight women with high cholesterol, eating three pears or three apples every day increased weight loss by nearly a pound, compared to women who ate little fruit. These same women had greater reductions in calorie intake and were more likely to feel satisfied after eating. The fruit-eating ladies also had greater decreases in blood glucose, compared to fruit slackers.

Pineapples

Pineapples are the second-richest source and leading fruit source of manganese, in addition to their other beneficial nutrients (see page 290). In particular, they contain the enzyme bromelain, known for its ability to reduce inflammatory processes in the body. A study involving inflammatory breast cancer cells exposed to bromelain found that apoptosis (cancer cell death) was markedly increased when the cells came in contact with the enzyme.

Plums and Prunes

Given your druthers, go with dried plums, a.k.a. prunes, over fresh, for their superior nutrition (see page 290). Prunes can help manage weight, as research has found that they do a better job of suppressing appetite, compared to other popular snack items such as low-fat cookies. Nutrients found in prunes may help control hormones that regulate appetite. Prune consumption is also associated with reduced fat that collects in the belly region and also with reductions in LDL cholesterol production in both animals and humans. They are rich in phenolic compounds and other nutrients that help build bone and maintain bone health. Last but not least, prunes promote digestive health and were found to be more palatable and more effective than psyllium for the treatment of mild to moderate constipation.

Raspberries

Raspberries, and their cousin blackberries, are a powerhouse of nutrition (see page 290). In a cancer cell study, black raspberries and their bioactive components significantly reduced the growth of human cervical cancer cells. Cell and animal research also support the cancer fighting, blood pressure–lowering, and inflammation-busting properties in both blackberries and red raspberries.

Sapodillas

Read about the many benefits of this tropical fruit on page 291. Young sapodilla fruit is very high in tannins, which impart a very astringent taste so typically this form is not as popular. However, because of the tannin content, young fruits are often boiled and the resulting juice is used as an effective treatment for diarrhea. Sapodillas are also rich in polyphenolic antioxidants, which were found in a cell study to have huge cancer cell–killing capacity for colon cancer.

Strawberries

Strawberries are a rich source of vitamins, minerals, and phytonutrients (see page 291). For some time now, cell and animal studies have supported the many benefits of consuming strawberries for heart and brain health. More recently, in a review study from the *Journal of Agriculture and Food Chemistry,* there is now human data that show that eating strawberries in both your immediate and long-term future will increase the amount of antioxidants you have on hand to do battle with disease. Anthocyanins, the pigment that makes strawberries red, boost antioxidant levels in the blood in as little as thirty minutes after eating them. After six weeks, strawberries reduced levels of inflammatory C-reactive protein and other markers of inflammation, such as IL-1 and tumor necrosis factor (TNF). Even more cool, strawberries may possess phytochemicals that offer antioxidant, anti-inflammatory, and direct effects on the brain itself in reducing cognitive deficits due to normal aging and dementia in older adults. Lastly, strawberries really shine when it comes to heart health. In a double-blind clinical study featured in the *British Journal of Nutrition,* obese adults who consumed the equivalent of 4 cups of strawberries via a strawberry powder concentrate for three weeks had greater reductions in total cholesterol and small HDL cholesterol particles (not the good kind) and increased LDL cholesterol particle size (the latest thinking is, you want your LDL particles *big!*), compared to the control group. Strawberries were found to help reduce risk of stroke and heart disease, even in an obese population.

Watermelon

Two cups of watermelon deliver more of the phytonutrient lycopene than does any other produce item. Watermelon is also an excellent source of vitamins A and C, and even its seeds are nutritious (see page 109). Want to spoil your appetite on purpose?

> Seedless watermelons came into existence about fifty years ago. However, you may find white "seeds" in them, which in actuality are really seed coats where the seed did not mature. Black mature seeds and seed coats are perfectly edible and good for you, and will never grow in your stomach (see page 109).

Like drinking water before a meal, eating a nice cold slice of watermelon has been found to tame that crazy hunger that promotes overeating. Try adding chunks of watermelon with a splash of watermelon juice to your humdrum water to create spa water! The white rind of watermelon is rich in the amino acid citrulline, which is a precursor of the artery-widening arginine. A recent study in obese subjects found that extracts of watermelon that contain these substances lowered ankle systolic and diastolic blood pressure readings.

BEST VEGETABLES

SNEAK-A-PEEK

Food (raw or cooked)	Serving
Asparagus	1 cup
Artichokes	1 cup
Beans	1 cup
Broccoli	1 cup
Carrots	1 cup
Corn	1 cup
*Garlic	1+ clove
Greens, Collard	2 cups
Kale	2 cups
Lettuce	2 cups
Mushrooms	1 cup
Okra	1 cup
Onions	1 medium
Peppers	1 cup
Potato	1 cup, or 1 medium baked
Pumpkin	1 cup
Spinach	2 cups
Squash (winter)	1 cup
Sweet potatoes	1 cup
Tomatoes	1 cup

*See page 256.

Honorable mentions: All others! There's no such thing as a bad vegetable!

What are vegetables and why should you eat them? I could take the easy way out and say, "Vegetables are whatever is not a fruit." From a botanical sense, I'm not far off. Basically, any part of a plant that is edible, such as stalks, leaves, roots, and rhizomes, constitutes a vegetable. Where the confusion lies is what we culinarily consider a vegetable: such foods as tomatoes, beans, and avocados. Vegetables are often divided up into the categories of dark green, red or orange, beans and peas, starchy, and "other." Each category brings something unique to the dinner table, as well as health benefits to your body. That's why no "best" vegetable list is worth the paper it was written on unless these groups are included!

Why should you eat them? Let me count the ways! First off, vegetables are the quintessential example of a nutrient-dense food. They contain lots of vitamins, minerals, and plant chemicals, all for very little calorie contribution. The Harvard-based Nurses' Health Study and Health Professionals Follow-up Study looked at the dietary habits of almost 110,000 men and women for fourteen years. What they found is that those who consumed higher than average daily intake of fruits and vegetables had lower chances of developing cardiovascular disease and having a heart attack or stroke. All of the big health associations agree that adding more vegetables to your diet is associated with healthier living.

HOW MUCH IS ENOUGH?

Depending on your age, gender, and level of activity, your daily vegetable recommendation can vary greatly. Refer to this MyPlate.gov chart to see what amount is right for you!

Daily Recommendation for Vegetables			
Age (years)	Children (cups/day)	Males (cups/day)	Females (cups/day)
2–3	1		
4–8	1½		
9–13		2½	2
14–18		3	2½
19–30		3	2½
31–50		3	2½
51+		2½	2

SOURCE: MyPlate.gov

Did you know? As mentioned in my discussion of fresh fruits, less than 6 percent of Americans are meeting all of the dietary guidelines, and the one area we are really falling down on is eating adequate amounts of produce. Looking at the following chart: From 1999 to 2009, we have cut our

Daily Recommendation for Vegetables by Type

Age (years)	Males (cups/week)					Females (cups/week)				
	Dark Green	Red/Orange	Legumes	Starchy	Other	Dark Green	Red/Orange	Legumes	Starchy	Other
2–3	½	2½	½	2	1½	½	2½	½	2	1½
4–8	1	3	½	3½	2½	1	3	½	3½	2½
9–13	1½	5½	1½	5	4	1½	4	1	4	3½
14–18	2	6	2	6	5	1½	5½	1½	5	4
19–30	2	6	2	6	5	1½	5½	1½	5	4
31–50	2	6	2	6	5	1½	5½	1½	5	4
51+	1½	5½	1½	5	4	1½	4	1	4	3½

vegetable and fruit production by nearly 60 pounds per person per year! If every person all of a sudden "got religion" and wanted to eat the amounts recommended in the MyPlate charts, our current rate of fruit and vegetable production would not be able to meet the demand. Let's create that need *now*!

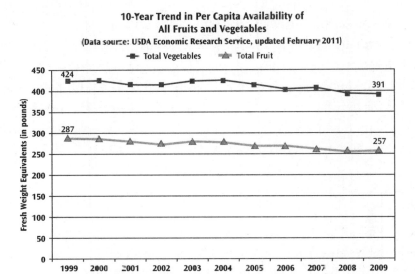

**10-Year Trend in Per Capita Availability of
All Fruits and Vegetables**
(Data source: USDA Economic Research Service, updated February 2011)

SOURCE: Alliance for Potato Research and Education

Asparagus

Turn to page 285 for the skinny on this skinny vegetable. Time to clear the air when it comes to the odor produced in pee by some asparagus. Theories abound about what causes it and why others can eat asparagus until the cows come home and not wrinkle a nose. Researchers from the Monell Chemical Senses Center in Philadelphia evaluated thirty-eight adult subjects who ate asparagus and then collected urine samples from them. They also collected urine samples from the same subjects on a day they did not eat asparagus. The goal was to see whether the subjects could detect which sample was from the day that asparagus was consumed. The authors of the study found that there were individual differences in subjects' ability to produce odor and also detect odor. And for those who had an inability to detect asparagus pee, it may be due to a variation (polymorphism) in a smell gene, called rs4481887. Translated? If you can smell it, other people may not be able to. If you can't smell it, others who have that polymorphism might be able to. Just eat the asparagus and don't worry about it, or bring spray with you.

Artichokes

Research in 2004 found artichoke hearts one of the highest-antioxidant vegetables on earth. Artichokes may protect against heart disease for those with abnormally high lipid levels. The soluble fiber and other nutrients in artichokes may not only choke off the ability of the liver to produce cholesterol, but simultaneously help pack it up and send it with a one-way ticket to the porcelain bowl. The antioxidants also slow down LDL cholesterol oxidation and keep the inside lining of arteries supple. Read more about the advantages of this prickly vegetable on page 132.

Beans

Beans count as meat equivalents and are also card-carrying members of the vegetable family, per the USDA MyPlate guidelines. If I had limited this list to "The Two Best Vegetables," the category of beans would be a top contender, for sure! Beans have almost everything you need for survival—fiber, iron, protein, and tons of other nutrients and phytochemicals (see page 286). The American Cancer Society, the American Institute for Cancer Research, the Academy of Nutrition and Dietetics, the American Diabetes Association, and the American Heart Association (to name a few) are organizations that encourage bean consumption to put a serious hurt on those free radicals in your body that try to cause trouble (heart disease, cancer, diabetes . . . you name it!). I feel so strongly about your getting this important vegetable group into your diet that I'm okay if you put the book down and check whether you have some in your cabinets. Go ahead—I'll wait.

Broccoli

Broccoli is a powerhouse of vitamins, minerals, and antioxidants (see page 45), yet *Men's Fitness* magazine declared it the second-most-hated food among men (after Brussels sprouts). Hey! They forgot to interview me! I would have shared simple and easy guy-friendly ways to prepare it, such as in a simple stir-fry or rolled into a frittata, or pan-roasted with Brussels sprouts (yes!) and onions in a balsamic glaze. Yikes, I've just drooled on the page—sorry. Anyhow, I would have also told them of a recent study where researchers in the journal *Clinical Epigenetics* found that the substance sulforaphane, found in broccoli, does the old one-two-punch on cancer cells by preventing them from multiplying and then strong-arming them into the body's cancer-cell disposal system.

Carrots

Carrots are the undisputed veggie leader when it comes to vitamin A content. One cup will meet your need for over six days! Carrots also deliver a nice hit of fiber and an assortment of vitamins and minerals (see page 287). Carrots are a type of vegetable that doesn't lose much in nutrition when you cook it. In fact, the body's ability to absorb beta-carotene may be enhanced when carrots are cooked, pureed, or juiced. And if you have picky kids, adding some carrot juice or puree into other foods they enjoy is a creative way of meeting their nutrition needs.

Corn

Corn has been leading a dual life! When it's fresh, it's considered a vegetable; and when it's dried, it is considered a grain. Either way, it is worthy of your digestive tract (see page 287). One of the health attributes of corn can be found in its resistant starch. Cornstarch is categorized as a resistant starch, which is considered a third type of fiber in addition to soluble and insoluble fiber. It "resists" digestion but still helps aid health by producing short-chain fatty acids in the digestive tract, specifically a kind called butyrate which may fight colon cancer. Resistant starch has also been found effective in helping to manage blood glucose, digestion, and weight.

> The average ear of corn has about eight hundred kernels, arranged in sixteen rows. There is one piece of silk for each kernel.

Garlic*

Why the asterisk? There is a debate among those culinary and nutrition experts in the world, about whether garlic counts as a vegetable or an herb. Garlic is in the Allium family and is closely related to onions, leeks, and scallions—all considered vegetables. But I can't in good conscience suggest you eat a cupful like the other veggies on this list. The World Health Organization suggests a clove a day for good health. I followed WHO's lead for serving size. Garlic contains the plant nutrients, such as allicin, alliin, and saponins, which researchers have found play a role in boosting immune function, lowering blood pressure and cholesterol, and fighting cancer. See page 160 for more about this beneficial member of the onion family. Researchers at Washington State University discovered that a compound in garlic called diallyl sulfide is one hundred times more effective than two leading antibiotics at fighting the *Campylobacter* bacterium, one of the most common causes of food poisoning. "Waiter— extra garlic, please!"

Collard Greens

Collard greens are a wonderful source of vitamins, minerals, and fiber (see page 7). Collards belong to the cruciferous family of veggies that also includes kale, broccoli, cabbage, and cauliflower—all known for their intolerance of cancer cells. Every time crucifers see cancer cells, they just want to hurt them . . . real bad. Next to kale, collards bring you the most vitamin K, which is important for blood clotting—unless you clot too much; then eating collards would not be a good thing to do.

Kale

Kale is delicious raw in salad or cooked. Like its cruciferous cousin collards, it is supernutritious (see page 7). Fruits and vegetables that are high in carotenoids, such as crucifers, may help lower the risk of cancers of the lung, esophagus, and mouth. Researchers also found that eating lots of cruciferous vegetables demonstrated reduced risk of developing breast cancer, which may be due to a group of plant nutrients called glucosinolates, which may slow down estrogen metabolism and protect cells from harmful mutations.

Lettuce

Dark green leafy lettuce has good nutrition value but romaine lettuce is the most nutritious (see page 189), and providing five times more vitamin C than iceberg. Adding a little bit of fat either from nuts or dressing helps with the absorption of its nutrients. Two cups of romaine supplies nearly 30 percent of your daily folate needs. Animal research found that when leafy green lettuce was added to the diet of mice, antioxidant levels improved, while lipid profiles improved as well. Barbara Rolls, PhD, at Penn State University, found that eating a salad before a main course helped reduce overall calorie consumption from the actual meal because of lettuce's ability to make one feel full.

Mushrooms

Mushrooms are low in calories and loaded with nutrition (see pages 14 and 20). They are the highest vegetarian source of vitamin D. Mushroom research is really mushrooming! You can almost name a major health challenge and mushrooms are all too happy to help. Cell, animal, and human studies suggest that mushrooms can help boost immunity, fight cancer, lower cholesterol and blood pressure, boost vitamin D levels, and manage weight and hunger. That's a mouthful. Mushrooms impart umami, a savory quality that is often called the fifth taste. Umami-rich foods also help fool the tongue that it's getting more of a salty taste, which is quite helpful in making lower-sodium diets more enjoyable!

Okra

Nutritious okra (see page 289) is notable for its high fiber. A cornerstone of Dr. David Jenkins' research at the University of Toronto is the use of viscous fibers from such vegetables as okra. He found that his portfolio diet rivaled first-line statin drugs in their ability to tame unruly cholesterol levels, without the potential side effects of statin drugs.

Onions

Among their other nutrients (see page 57), onions contain a plant flavonoid called quercetin, which has amazing antioxidant properties. Some studies have found that quercetin squashes free radicals and prevents them from doing damage to the body, especially to LDL cholesterol, preventing it from turning into the more dangerous oxidized form. Speaking of heart health, onions also keep blood slippery and reduce the possibility of deadly clots that can lead to strokes and heart attacks. Onions absolutely hate ulcer-producing bacteria *H. pylori* and get a kick out of stopping it from growing. The quercetin in onions has also been attributed to increasing bone density in rats, which may translate to lessening the chances of developing osteoporosis in humans.

Peppers

Bell peppers are in the same family as chile peppers, but have a much milder flavor—especially the red, orange, and yellow varieties. Peppers are a great source of vitamin C, which helps our body heal from wounds, fights infection, and protect the cells from damage. See pages 43 and 44 for the additional benefits of sweet and hot peppers.

> Only green peppers were grown and popular in recipes until the 1980s, and now all different colors of bell peppers are grown, including white, yellow, red, orange, and brown!

Potato

Potatoes are an excellent source of vitamin C and potassium, and a good source of vitamin B_6. What's amazing to me is how many "experts" pin the obesity epidemic on the lowly potato and are clamoring for its removal from the American diet. As you can see from the graph, there has been a slow but steady decrease in the consumption of potato products over the past decade or so. Potatoes are an excellent source of potassium—yet only 3 percent of Americans are meeting their potassium needs. Shouldn't we be

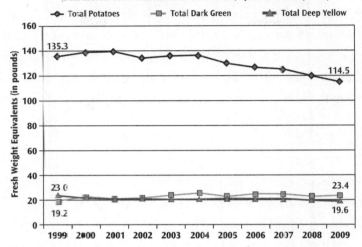

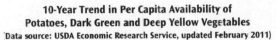

**10-Year Trend in Per Capita Availability of
Potatoes, Dark Green and Deep Yellow Vegetables**
Data source: USDA Economic Research Service, updated February 2011)

SOURCE: Alliance for Potato Research and Education

clamoring for more, not less, potato consumption? The potato has evolved beyond the vat of boiling oil, and so should our cuisine. Potatoes can be enjoyed in so many ways, but I always recommend that you should leave its skin on for maximum nutrition and health benefit. (See page 53 for the surprising benefits of potato chips.)

Pumpkin

Pumpkin offers a wealth of healthy benefits (see page 6). Pumpkin, pumpkin seeds, and pumpkin seed oil have been used for centuries as a folk remedy to help with a variety of health conditions. Pumpkin may help with controlling blood glucose, according to animal studies, and pumpkin seeds and its oil may be beneficial in controlling swollen prostates and decreasing the risk of prostate cancer.

Spinach

Spinach may be the supreme leader of this list, as it appears more than any other vegetable in other lists in this book (see page 291 for a full lineup of its benefits). There are so many health conditions that spinach may offer help in, such as cancer, heart disease, bone health, diabetes, and the list goes on. An interesting human study found that moderate consumption of spinach offers protection to our very DNA by preventing oxidation. This could have profound implications for cancer prevention and slowing down the aging process. Also in the same study, folate increased, while inflammation markers such as homocysteine dropped markedly.

Squash

Cubed, baked butternut squash is an excellent source of fiber and vitamins A, B_6, and C, and a good source of folate, iron, magnesium, niacin, potassium, thiamine, and vitamin E. When it comes to plant nutrients for eye health, beta-carotene and lutein always take center stage. But always in their shadows is another plant nutrient called zeaxanthin, of which winter squashes are a rich source. An animal study found that higher concentrations of zeaxanthin in the retina of the eye offered more protection from photo damage, while retinas with low concentrations had suffered severe light damage.

Sweet Potatoes

Sweet potatoes make a great first baby food and should be enjoyed throughout the life cycle. Regular sweet potatoes are an amazing source of nutrients (see page 6), including beta-carotene, but purple varieties offer even more diverse plant nutrients, such as anthocyanins—specifically cyanidin and peonidin—which researchers from Kansas State discovered have strong anticancer properties. Purple sweet potatoes have been found to be quite effective in reducing exercise-induced oxidative damage and may offer powerful protection against cognitive deficits that lead to brain disorders.

Tomatoes

Americans eat between 22 and 24 pounds of tomatoes and tomato products per person per year! Tomatoes come in many different varieties and can be found at the store fresh or canned in many forms, including whole, chopped, puree, sauce, and paste. Cooked tomatoes are even healthier than fresh; see page 217. The American Cancer Society estimated that there will be 240,890 cases of prostate cancer in 2011, which makes it the most common of all cancers diagnosed. Tomatoes and tomato products are packed with the antioxidant lycopene, as well as vitamins A and C, which may help fight prostate cancer.

> The largest tomato on record weighed 7 pounds 12 ounces and was grown in Oklahoma in 1986. That's as big as a baby! The farmer who grew it sliced it up and served twenty-one sandwiches! I was not invited . . .

BEST PROTEIN FOODS

SNEAK-A-PEEK

Food	Serving
Beef*	3 ounces
Eggs (white)**	3 egg whites
Milk**	1 cup
Soy*	1 cup
Whey*	1 ounce

*The protein digestibility-corrected amino acid score (PDCAAS) for isolated soy is the same as the protein in eggs, whey, and milk. Whole soy foods and beef scored lower on the PDCAAS scale.
**Highest in PDCAAS

Honorable mentions: Poultry, nuts, beans, grains

What is protein and what are the best protein foods? Protein is needed to build and repair muscle tissue, but it's also integral to cranking out enzymes and hormones that help support every cell and system in our body, from digestion to immunity. Protein is made up of individual building blocks called amino acids. And if needed in a pinch, they can supply the body with energy, too.

Protein can be found in both animal and plant sources. Although they differ in quality, both kinds of proteins can meet the needs of the average American. There are twenty amino acids that humans need each and every day, nine of which are considered indispensible yet which cannot be manufactured by the body. This is only a concern with diets that are made up entirely of plant-based proteins. Vegans, who consume no animal products, must be careful to include complementary proteins in their diet (e.g., grains and beans). When combined, these plant proteins supply all nine indispensible amino acids. Other forms of vegetarianism are not a concern because even the smallest amount of meat, fish, or dairy products added to incomplete plant proteins makes them complete.

Did you know? The quality and timing of protein are important for those who are more performance and athletically inclined. Here, I have used the internationally accepted method of ranking protein quality, called the protein digestibility-corrected amino acid score (PDCAAS): Proteins are ranked based on whether they contain all of the indispensible amino acids and also by their rate of digestibility. For athletes, sports nutrition experts recommend that a high-quality protein be consumed within two hours of exercise, a period of time called the anabolic window, which favors optimal protein synthesis.

HOW MUCH IS ENOUGH?

Level of activity	Recommended Daily Protein Intake (per kg of body weight)
Sedentary adults	0.8 g/kg
Recreational athletes*	1.0 g/kg
Endurance athletes	1.2–1.4 g/kg
Ultraendurance athletes	1.2–2.0 g/kg
Strength athletes	1.2–2.0 g/kg

*Low to moderate training volume and intensity.
Excerpted from *Nutrition for Sports and Exercise* by Marie Dunford and J. Andrew Doyle, Wadsworth Publishing, 2011

Beef

Sarcopenia is a condition of muscle wasting that occurs as early as the mid-forties, which is estimated to increase the risk of disability later in life by three- to fourfold. The current dietary reference intake of 0.8 g of protein per kilogram of body weight may not be enough, according to some protein researchers, to stave off this condition. A 3-ounce portion of beef provides about 25 g of protein (51 percent of the DV). Another study found that consuming 4 ounces of lean beef protein each day can help enhance muscle development by 50 percent and delay the onset of sarcopenia or loss of muscle. Eating at least 15 g of essential amino acids at each meal, equivalent to 4 ounces of a high-quality protein, such as lean meat, may help maintain muscle mass and provide strength to lead an active lifestyle. To read more about the benefits of beef, turn to page 66.

Eggs

Don't get the yolk? Boy, are you missing out. Eggs whites are only half the story, as yolks provide almost half the protein in eggs, plus most of the nutrients (see page 287)! And starting the day with a few whole eggs may help you on the scale later on, as research suggests that the protein in eggs provides satiety and can spell calorie savings at the end of the day, due to reduced cravings for snacks plus a smaller appetite overall.

Milk

Milk is an excellent source of numerous vitamins and minerals (see page 289). A variety of factors contribute to increased risk of osteoporosis, including low calcium intake, low physical activity, being overweight or too thin, and genetics, to name a few. Besides ingesting adequate calcium to build up bone stores when we are young, consuming calcium along with other cofactors that can aid in absorption is equally important. The greatest contributor of calcium to the American diet is dairy, which also provides vitamin D (thanks to fortification) as well as other conutrients that help drive calcium into bones. Of particular interest here is the role of bioactive protein components that naturally occur in milk, which enhance calcium absorption. Dairy also contains a unique blend of slow-acting (casein) and fast-acting (whey) proteins—an ideal combo to ingest postexercise, as whey supplies an immediate source of amino acids to aid in muscle recovery, while casein helps slow down the rate of muscle breakdown.

Soy

Isolated soy protein powder can go head to head with some of the big boys mentioned here; however, whole soybean foods, though containing all of the nine indispensible amino acids, don't score as high on the PDCAAS chart. That said, cooked soybeans are supernutritious (see page 291), and still provide a decent dose of protein.

Whey

Whey and casein are the two major proteins found in milk. During the cheese-making process, whey is separated from the cheese curds when enzymes are added to the milk. Then the liquid whey is dried and sold in powder form. Historically, the liquid whey would be fed to animals or discarded. Now whey is valued as one the highest protein sources on earth! A serving of whey is an excellent source of protein and a good source of calcium. The amino acid profile of whey protein closely resembles that of skeletal muscle in the body. In fact, whey provides an excellent amount of branched-chain amino acids (BCAAs) vital for muscle repair. Whey is also rich in the amino acid glutamine, which helps reduce muscle breakdown and bolsters glutathione production in muscles and the liver, which in turn enhances immune function. A double-blind, randomized clinical trial of ninety overweight or obese subjects found that the group that consumed 56 g of whey protein per day for twenty-three weeks reduced their body weight by an average of 4 pounds and body fat by an average of 5 pounds, while also reducing their waist circumference and the hunger-stimulating hormone ghrelin. The interesting thing about the study is none of the groups were instructed to change anything about their diets.

BEST SNACK FOODS

SNEAK-A-PEEK

Food	Serving
Bowl of whole-grain cereal with low-fat or skim milk	Varies, depending on the cereal. Have at least ½ cup of milk on it.
Dairy	1 cup
Nuts and fruit Nut bars	1 ounce 1 bar
Popcorn	3 cups
Prunes	½ cup

Honorable mentions: Beans, fruit, vegetables, low fat and low-sodium lunch meats

What is healthy snacking? First, some points of clarity. *Anything* you eat can be considered a "snack." That can be a good thing or a problem, depending on the impact of snacking on your total calorie and nutrient intake in the day. Snack foods that tend to be overconsumed are potato chips and nachos, crackers, cookies, pastries, and nuts.

So, is snacking a good or a bad thing to do? Well, that depends on the individual and what is considered a snack. For some, snacking helps stabilize their blood sugar and manage their appetite so they aren't ravenous by the time the next meal rolls around. For others, snacking triggers disordered eating whereby portion control and mindful eating all goes out the window. The research is mixed on the value of snacking; however, a larger study of over eleven thousand adults, featured in the *Journal of the Academy of Dietetics and Nutrition,* found that snacking has a more positive than negative impact on the quality of our diet. When compared to the Department of Agriculture's Healthy Eating Index 2005 (HEI), snacking up to four times a day was associated with higher total HEI scores. The researchers found that more servings of fruits, whole grains, and milk were consumed via snacking—but so were fats and sodium. Interestingly, an inverse relationship between snacking frequency and vegetable, meat, and bean intake was observed. However, fewer overall calories from solid fat, alcohol, and added sugars were observed, which to me, is a good thing. Bottom line: Snackers seem to enjoy a more nutrient-dense diet. Even when it comes to chips, healthier choices are becoming available, thanks to mandatory trans fats labeling. Besides trans fats virtually disappearing from snacks, the reduction of partially hydrogenated fats has not reduced the amount of saturated fats in chips, but we have seen saturated fats go up in cookies. The other good news is that rolling out snack-size portions, such as the 100-calorie packs, has made a difference in calorie consumption, according to the latest research. (That is assuming you eat just one pack for a snack—two if you are a bigger guy like me!)

I already know that some of you out there may be asking, "Why didn't broccoli make it on your list?" I can't imagine anyone would argue that raw crudités and such are automatic implied members of this list, but I wanted to move beyond the obvious and tackle the other category where it might be harder to tell what's better: Corn chip or potato chip? Rice cake or cracker?

Did you know? A study of college kids found that whether they considered a food a "snack" or a "meal" influenced their eating behavior. In essence, if the food was considered to be just a snack, they ate considerably more calories of it, compared to if they thought of the same item as a meal. A recent study found that adolescents consume a quarter of their calories as snacks.

Shocker Food!

Controlling appetite is governed by many different factors and one of the most commonly overlooked influencers is that of chewing, a.k.a. orosensory stimulation. Chewing gum has often been heralded for its ability to suppress cravings for smoking, as well as those for sweets or other high-calorie snacks. Sixty participants were asked to eat a lunch provided for them and rate their hunger, appetite, and cravings for sweet and salty snacks every hour after the meal, until they returned three hours later for a snack. They did this same routine on four separate occasions. After two of the lunches, participants were asked to chew gum for fifteen minutes on every hour for the next three hours, until they were served a snack. A reduction in snack intake was observed, plus their ratings for hunger, appetite, and cravings for snacks diminished.

Bowl of Cereal

We often think of breakfast cereal as only being for breakfast. But it's also a superconvenient and delicious snack choice, especially when combined with skim milk. In fact, cereal and milk is the number one way that Americans take in ten essential vitamins and minerals for breakfast. Ready-to-eat cereal has fewer calories than many typical breakfast items, and did you know that cereal eaters consume less fat, less cholesterol, and more fiber than non-cereal eaters? But as you might imagine, not all cereals are created equal. Look for ones that have what I call the 5+5 factor: at least 5 g of fiber and at least 5 g of protein. Fiber and protein have a tremendous influence on appetite. Pouring on ½ cup of milk gives you an additional 4 g of protein to boost this snack combo to 9 g. That amount of protein helps take the edge off your appetite. Breakfast aside, a bowl of cereal and skim milk after an athletic event was found to be as effective in stimulating muscle recovery as a sports drink. A study showed that when cereal was used in place of a normal evening snack in seventy overweight subjects, small reductions in waist circumference and calorie intake were reduced after six weeks, compared with baseline. Cereal, in the form of cereal bars, improved alertness in those who ate them as an evening snack, according to a study. So, think outside the cereal box—cereal's not just for breakfast anymore!

Dairy

Dairy products have been a popular choice for snacking as far back as anyone can remember. Whether it's low-fat milk, chocolate milk, yogurt, kefir, or cheese, all dairy is nutrient dense and supplies lots of hunger-busting protein, along with other vital nutrients. Check 'em out! For example, 1½ ounces of Cheddar cheese is an excellent source of calcium and phosphorus, and a good source of riboflavin, vitamins A and B_{12}, and zinc. Dairy products, mainly due to their proteins, satisfy hunger and give more of a sense of fullness. Research shows that snacking on dairy can have a positive impact on calorie intake and body weight, which can be achieved within (not in addition to) the recommendation of three dairy servings a day. Milk proteins also have a positive effect on managing blood glucose.

A premeal snack of dairy may also be helpful in controlling the glycemic response to carbohydrate contained within that meal.

Nuts and Fruit

The perfect blend! Mixing almonds, peanuts, pecans, pistachios, and walnuts together might be an ideal snack mix, as all have demonstrated the ability to stop hunger in its tracks. Nuts are a goldmine of nutrition (see the nutrient contents chart beginning on page 285 to discover the nutrition value of nuts), which benefits heart health and the waistline, though one would think that because they are so high in fat, nuts would be more associated with needing to buy larger pants. Several studies show no weight gain when nuts are consumed in moderate portions regularly; indeed, some studies even show an inverse relationship between eating nuts and sporting a muffin top. Nutrition and science experts feel this may be due to the high-satiety effect of nuts' protein, fiber, and fat, and the effects of chewing. Some studies even suggest that the fats in nuts are poorly absorbed. In combination with fruits, your snack gets even better: A randomized study investigated the effects of a fruit and nut snack bar on body measurements, lipid panel, and blood pressure in ninety-four overweight adults. Participants were asked to add two bars daily to their existing diet for eight weeks. The bars totaled about 340 calories. Weight did not increase for the intervention group, suggesting that the bars may have provided satiety; that is, the participants consumed lower quantities of other foods.

Popcorn

Everyone knows that popcorn, without all of that oily butter, salt, or other imaginative toppings, is a pretty healthy whole-grain option. But what is most surprising is that popcorn contains polyphenols that rival the amount found in many of the healthiest fruits and vegetables. Lead researcher Joe Vinson, PhD, reported at the 2012 American Chemical Society convention, held in San Diego, that polyphenol content is richer in a serving of popcorn because it is not diluted as you would find in fruits and vegetables, which contain about 90 percent water. And don't throw away the hulls that are left at the bottom of the popcorn (my fave!)—those have the most polyphenols and fiber of the entire kernel! For comparison's sake, a serving of popcorn contains roughly 300 mg of polyphenols per serving compared to 160 mg per serving for some of the top-ranking fruits and vegetables.

One of the consequences of not eating enough whole grains that are rich in fiber is the increased risk of developing diverticular disease of the bowel. Many who are diagnosed with diverticulosis are often instructed by their physician to avoid such foods as popcorn for fear that one of the kernels may get lodged in an outpouching of the colon called a diverticulum. Ironically, a study in 2008 of nearly forty-eight thousand men found that, over an eighteen-year period of time, there was an inverse association between eating popcorn and other "concerning" foods, such as nuts, and the risk of developing diverticulitis (the inflamed version of diverticulosis)! Furthermore, for those who had diverticulosis, no associations were seen between including popcorn, corn, or nuts and an aggravation of their existing diverticulitis. The authors concluded that the recommendation to avoid popcorn should be reconsidered.

Prunes

A randomized study of forty-five adults found that those who snacked on prunes before eating a meal consumed less dessert and ate fewer calories at the meal. Additionally, the participants reported that they didn't feel as hungry in between the time they ate the snack and had a meal. The researchers behind the study felt that the sensation of satiety was most likely due to the fiber content of prunes. Different snack foods were compared for their effect on satiety, blood glucose, and hormone response. Nineteen adult women fasted and then ate four different snacks that included prunes, cookies, white bread, and water. All of the foods, but not the water, supplied about 240 calories and about the same fat, protein, and carbohydrate, but contained differing amounts of fiber and sugar. Subjects were more satisfied with the prunes versus the cookies. There wasn't a difference in how much was eaten at the meal they consumed after having their snack; however, the prunes resulted in lower glucose and insulin and did not affect satiety-regulating hormones as the cookies did.

CHAPTER 10

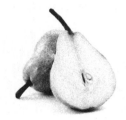

Top Performers

7 BEST PRE- AND POSTWORKOUT FOODS

SNEAK-A-PEEK

Food	Serving
Bananas	1 large
Cherries (raw) Cherries (dried)	1 cup ½ cup
Chocolate milk	1 cup
Kefir	1 cup
Oatmeal (cooked)	1 cup
Peanut butter	1 tablespoon
Raisins	½ cup

Featuring dietary recommendations from sports nutrition experts Nancy Clark, MS, RD, CSSD, author of several publications including *Nancy Clark's Sports Nutrition Guidebook*, and Jan Dowell, MS, MES, RD, CSSD, associate professor at Benedictine University in Lisle, Illinois.

Honorable mentions: Preworkout: Grains such as bread, bagels, pancakes, waffles, and pretzels; berries; dark chocolate; watermelon; and sports drinks. Postworkout: Carbohydrate replacement drinks, low-fat dairy, fatty fish, lean poultry and lean meat, eggs, whey, soy, fruits and vegetables, whole grains, vegetable juice, and beer!

Best food groups: Whole grains, fruit, vegetables, lean proteins, low-fat dairy

Why is it important to fuel before, during, and after exercise? Eating a proper diet at the appropriate time is not just for serious athletes. Whoever exercises or trains in any capacity should fuel their body optimally to perform their best.

> **Pre-event:** Many nutrition experts agree that the lines between pre- and postevent workout foods are a bit blurred, but feel that a balance of carbohydrate, protein, and fat is important for muscle development, repair, and recovery. Carbohydrate is the preferred source of fuel for active muscles but it's not a bad idea to add a bit of healthy fat and protein before the event, to have it on board to begin the repair process and to prevent hunger and keep your mind on training or the race. Low-fiber foods are recommended pre-event because they can cause less bloating during physical activity—the time to fiber up is *after*, not before exercise! Avoid the following prior to exercising: large doses of caffeine; carbonated beverages; high-fiber cereals; beans; gassy vegetables such as cabbage, broccoli, onions, and garlic; fried foods; and large quantities of dried fruit and juices.
>
> **Event:** During exercise, the preferred source of fuel by muscles is carbohydrate, in the form of glucose. It is important to supply your body with glucose via sports drinks, bars, gels, and such if you will be exercising intensely for longer than thirty minutes; otherwise, don't worry too much about using them. The amount of carbohydrate you need varies, depending on your weight and type of training you do. It's best to consult with a sports nutrition specialist for specific recommendations. Visit www.eatright.org to find board-certified sports dietitian (CSSD) in your area.
>
> **Postevent:** Athletes, and others serious about health and training performance goals, want to ensure their recovery is optimized, via superior nutrition strategies. Exercise depletes energy stores in the muscle after a

hard workout, so it is important to know which foods enhance recovery, including restoring glycogen levels in the muscle. Muscle glycogen (the storage form of glucose) is the main fuel used during intense exercise and is also important during endurance exercise. A mix of carbohydrate and protein is particularly important for muscle repair. "Protein prior to an event probably doesn't matter unless the person is going to be doing a long event or training. Including protein afterward is essential," says Jan Dowell, MS, MHS, RD, CSSD. Recovery choices should include lots of fluids and nutrient and antioxidant-rich foods so as to enhance repair and diminish inflammation. "I also suggest a postevent snack that is salty, to help meet needs related to sodium replacement. Besides, many endurance athletes get tired of sweets after a long event," says Dowell.

Did you know? A review of research regarding nutritional strategies to optimize postexercise recovery found that the best timing for postworkout fuel is within one to two hours following a workout, ideally consuming that fuel within thirty minutes.

Shocker Food!

In 1882, a sweet cracker made from graham flour (unsifted whole wheat flour) was named after Reverend Sylvester Graham, who promoted the use of whole grains. "Graham crackers are a whole-grain, crunchy, and slightly sweet snack that goes really well with peanut butter for a change of pace from yet another granola bar," says Nancy Clark, MS, RD CSSD. Try making mini PBJs with graham crackers and 100 percent fruit jam. Pop in one or two, ideally one to two hours before a workout.

Bananas

"Bananas are an all-natural, prewrapped energizer that's filled with potassium and carbs to give muscles what they need," says Clark. See page 286 for more about the nutritional benefits of this fruit.

Of all fruits, bananas seem to be the most popular among Americans—an average of 33 pounds per person are eaten each year!

Cherries

The anthocyanins in cherries are known to decrease muscle soreness and also support heart health. Montmorency cherry juice and tart red cherry juice have been shown to reduce muscle damage and soreness caused by intense strength workouts and running. Turn to page 188 to learn more about cherries.

Chocolate Milk

Low-fat or fat-free chocolate milk is an effective, low-cost recovery beverage. Milk has a unique nutrient package, supplying nine essential nutrients (see page 222) and costing only about a quarter per serving. Chocolate milk has been found to have an ideal ratio of carbohydrate to protein for optimal postworkout recovery. A 2006 study found that it is also an excellent fuel between two exercise sessions. A 2009 study confirmed these results and showed chocolate milk is indeed an optimal beverage for endurance athletes.

> In 2011, Americans drank more than 3,522 million pounds of low-fat, flavored milk.

Kefir

Kefir is packed with nutrients (see page 224), is so portable, and doesn't require a spoon to eat, either! Low in fat and just the right amount of carbohydrates, kefir, consumed with fruit, is a perfect snack after a tough workout to replenish energy stores and encourage muscle growth and repair. The rigors and physical stress of training and competing in events can take its toll on the immune system of endurance athletes. Cultured dairy products, such as kefir, provide friendly bacteria that assist with boosting immune cells and benefit the digestive and upper respiratory tract and skin health, too. A Japanese animal study found that fermented milk reduced muscle damage after prolonged exercise, which the authors attributed to the increased antioxidant capacity of the muscles.

Oatmeal

"I love oatmeal because it is a more slowly digested carb for sustained energy," says Clark. In fact, a small study conducted at the Noll Physiological Research Center at Penn State compared a sweetened rolled-oat cereal with a sweetened oat flour cereal for its effect on endurance in athletes. The same subjects tried both cereals and were exercised to exhaustion. The athletes were able to exercise 16 percent longer when they ate the rolled-oat cereal. See page 160 to read more about oats.

Peanut Butter

"I like peanut butter—for healthy fats that fight inflammation, protein to build and repair muscles, and a vast assortment of vitamins," says Clark. For a full profile of this versatile legume, see page 28. A spoonful of peanut butter is a popular postworkout eat for a reason. Peanuts are a rich source of the polyphenol resveratrol (especially in the skin), which puts a serious hurt on inflammation. In fact, natural peanut butters contain more resveratrol than blended butters, according to a Spanish study. Experts say postworkout meals should definitely contain some carbohydrate and protein, but fat is important component of them, too, as long as the portion is moderate. Peanut and nut butters provide healthy fats, protein, fiber, many minerals, and convenience. "Obviously, peanut butter is my ultimate favorite sports food because it is yummy, satiating, comfortable for me to digest, and a source of protein," says Clark.

Raisins

A small (hand-size) box of raisins provides 34 g of carbohydrate, plus a broad array of nutrients (see page 245). Long distance cyclists and runners really enjoy using sports jelly beans and sports gels. But in side-by-side tests, cyclists and runners performed every bit as good training with raisins (which are better for you). Besides, raisins contain resveratrol, an effective anti-inflammatory phytochemical that can aid in repairing cells damaged from intense exercise. Raisins were shown to be a cost-effective fueling strategy over pricey sports gels.

THANKS FOR THE MEMORIES:
7 BEST MEMORY-BOOSTING FOODS

SNEAK-A-PEEK

Food	Serving
Blueberries	1 cup
Coffee	1 cup
Eggs	1
Concord grape juice Wine	8 ounces 5 ounces
Olive oil	1 tablespoon
Soybeans	1 cup
Turmeric	1 teaspoon

Honorable mentions: Strawberries, walnuts, whole grains, nuts, citrus

Best food groups: Fruits, vegetables, whole grains, lean proteins, nuts and seeds, low-fat dairy

What are memory-boosting foods? Forgetting someone's name, where you left your car keys, or even what day it is, can happen to the best of us. It's just a fact of life. That sort of thing happens more frequently as we get older as a normal part of the aging process. The good news is keeping both physically and mentally active keeps the mind sharp and senility at bay. What clogs the arteries that feed the heart can also block the arteries that feed the brain. Researchers have narrowed down the nutrients that seem to play a role in promoting healthy brain function. Foods have also been linked to decreased development of dementia and/or Alzheimer's disease. Nutrients of interest include caffeine, choline, curcumin, folic acid, omega-3s, polyphenols, and vitamins B_{12} and C.

Did you know? A diet rich in antioxidants helps promote memory and brain function. Antioxidant-rich foods tend to be easy to find in the produce section. Just let your eyes lead you to what's richly colored . . . naturally, of course! Dark greens, broccoli, sweet potatoes, and berries, for instance, are loaded with antioxidants.

Blueberries

At only 80 calories per cup, blueberries are an excellent source of vitamins and minerals (see page 286). Researchers found that this berry helped improve memory tasks in people at risk for dementia. In addition, blueberries' high flavonoid content has been found to help short- and long-term memory. Seventeen studies support the role of blueberries in improving memory and cognitive function in both animals and humans. You would be smart to remember to eat them!

Coffee

There aren't a whole lot of vitamin and minerals in a cup of Joe, but that doesn't mean that coffee doesn't deliver. What you will find in each cup is caffeine and the plant antioxidants chlorogenic acids, which have been found to battle Parkinson's and heart disease, among other health obstacles. In several animal and human studies, coffee consumption or components of coffee such as caffeine and polyphenols were associated with improved memory in both young and older adults. Regular coffee consumption was also found to be heart healthy and may reduce the risk of diabetes by up to 30 percent.

Eggs

Although the whites are a great lean protein source, in this case, the yolk is what makes eggs a great memory-boosting food. Eggs are an terrific source of a variety of nutrients (see page 287). Those that affect cognitive function include choline, folate, and vitamin B_{12}. In a study of 1,391 subjects who did not have dementia, it was found that those who had higher choline intake in their diet did better on memory tests.

Concord Grape Juice

Concord grape juice is rich in the same polyphenols and resveratrol that you'd find in wine. A university of Cincinnati double-blind, placebo-controlled study found that Concord grape juice improved the memory and cognitive functioning of older adult subjects who consumed the juice every day for twelve weeks. Read more about the virtues of grape juice on page 245.

Olive Oil

Olive oil is rich in monounsaturated fats and contains a host of polyphenol nutrients that may help lower cholesterol and inflammation and fight many different diseases (see page 160). The Mediterranean diet has been associated with better cognitive function and memory, believed to be due in part to its polyphenol content. A study of elderly subjects found a relationship between olive oil intake and better short- and long-term memory; and a three-city study in France found that those who had a higher consumption of olive oil had better visual memory than did those who consumed less.

Soybeans

Research in both animal and human studies found that soy can improve memory and cognition. Soy contains phosphatidylserine, which was shown in a Japanese human study to improve memory of those who had memory complaints. See page 161 for the many other healthful advantages of soy.

Turmeric

The curcumin in turmeric is a well-studied substance known to be the most potent anti-inflammatory in the plant kingdom. Several studies ranging from cell to animal and to human have demonstrated the memory and cognitive enhancing benefits of curcumin in both healthy and even cognitively challenged subjects, such as those with Alzheimer's disease. See page 206 for more about turmeric.

SWEET DREAMS ARE MADE OF THESE: 7 BEST FOODS FOR ZZZZ

SNEAK-A-PEEK

Food	Serving
Cherry juice	1 cup
Chicken	3 ounces
Salmon (cooked)	3 ounces
Pumpkin seeds	1 ounce
Lettuce	2 cups
Milk	1 cup
Walnuts	1 ounce

Honorable mentions: Potatoes and high-carbohydrate foods

Best food groups: Grains, fruits, vegetables, dairy

What foods help promote sleep and why? According the CDC, the lack of sleep is now considered a "public health epidemic." Sleep can be negatively influenced by many different factors, from medical illness to side effects of drugs to simply having a lot on your mind. Before trying to remedy your sleep deficit on your own, make sure you investigate what may be behind your sleep difficulties and seek proper professional attention. It could save you time, money, and many more sleepless nights.

Prescription and over-the-counter sleep aids don't address the root cause of a sleep disorder. They are a temporary fix until the driving force behind the problem can be addressed. Diet can play a major role in influencing sleep, from providing something as simple as occupancy in your gut so you don't wake up from a rumbling tummy, to essential nutrients that govern your sleep center. The key nutrients that govern sleep are the

B vitamins, calcium, magnesium, the amino acid tryptophan, and the brain chemical melatonin, which can be produced from tryptophan or even consumed in many common foods.

Did you know? It's recommended to have a small bedtime snack that contains a carbohydrate plus a little protein, no sooner than an hour before bedtime. It is believed that this small, nutrient-balanced snack causes the brain to produce serotonin that helps calm you and lets you drift off to la-la land. Besides heeding the dietary add-in advice from this section, it would be wise to make sure you address this list of sleep stealers first!

- **Staying up late because you want to:** Not getting enough sleep every night can cause you to eat more and feel hungrier, which is another reason it's important to get in the recommended zzzz per night. Skipping out on sleep causes an imbalance of the hormones leptin and ghrelin; this imbalance increases hunger and decreases satiety cues.
- **Eating large:** Also, eating a large meal after not sleeping well the night before was found to increase grogginess in a group of young men, where their driving skills were being assessed. Those men who ate a big lunch after having had fewer than five hours of sleep experienced more unintentional lane drifting than did those who ate a smaller meal. Friends don't let friends eat big and drive!
- **Being overweight:** If you're overweight, lose weight for better sleep. A randomized controlled study found that those who cut their calories and lost weight had vast improvements in obstructive sleep apnea. It's also a vicious cycle—being overweight interrupts restful sleep; interrupting restful sleep contributes to obesity.
- **Avoid stimulants:** Some people have more sensitivity to caffeinated food and beverages than do others. Ironically, my mother-in-law actually finds caffeinated coffee helps her sleep better at night—go figure. But for many, caffeine works as a mild stimulant that causes jitters and gets the brain working into overdrive. If you must have caffeine, make sure you have it no closer than two to three hours to bedtime, as it takes that long for caffeine to begin clearing from your system. Foods and beverages that contain the most caffeine include

coffee, green and black tea, energy drinks, caffeinated sodas such as cola and root beer, and chocolate. Even over-the-counter meds such as Excedrin may keep you up at night. The nicotine in cigarettes can also interrupt sleep.

- **Avoid alcohol before bedtime:** A Spanish study found that subjects' melatonin levels increased when they drank beer, and so did their antioxidant levels. They also found the higher the alcohol percentage, the higher the melatonin and antioxidant status. At first glance, this sounds like a fun answer to a sleep problem. Not so fast! Research shows that a drink or two may help you get to sleep but is disruptive for restful REM (rapid eye movement) sleep.

- **Eat one but don't be a (couch) potato:** Just starting a simple walking routine may be enough to bolster sleep by better management of weight and producing more of the sleep-promoting hormone serotonin. Engaging in more strenuous physical activity right before bedtime is often frowned upon by sleep experts. However, researchers from the University of South Carolina found that men who exercised as close as 30 minutes before bedtime did not experience impaired sleep.

Supplement it? The natural sleep formulas on the market may be worth a try before graduating to an OTC aid or seeking a prescription. A study of long-term care residents found that those who received a supplement containing 225 mg of magnesium, 5 mg of melatonin, and 11 mg of zinc slept better than those who weren't on the supplement. Research on the effectiveness of the herb valerian root is mixed but many feel they get more restful sleep when they take it. A double-blind, placebo-controlled study found that those who took a supplement containing GABA and 5-hydroxytrytophane went to sleep quicker and stayed asleep longer, compared to the control group.

Cherry Juice

Three separate studies have looked at the melatonin content of tart cherries and have established this fruit as one of the top melatonin-containing foods that may prove beneficial in improving sleep quality and duration. In the form of juice, cherries contain more sleep-promoting melatonin.

Shocker Food! ─────────

Eating some carbohydrates before bedtime is one of the best fuels for cranking out sleep-promoting serotonin. But don't have fatty fries or chips. Simple eat some leftover baked potato or pop one into the microwave for a few minutes until it's done, and top with salsa (not too spicy), accompanied by a glass of milk. Potatoes and milk contain potassium, which may prevent leg cramps and calm restless legs, as well as lower blood pressure.

Chicken

We always think of the Thanksgiving turkey as the item being most responsible for lulling us into a state of unconsciousness after the big feast, but to tell the truth, it may be more from the carb overload from the meal than from the tryptophan in turkey. Besides, chicken rules the roost when it comes to tryptophan content, anyway. Tryptophan helps produce serotonin, which in turn makes us feel more relaxed and sleepy. See page 17 for more nutritional benefits of chicken.

Salmon

Along with many other nutrients (see page 291), salmon is an excellent source of omega-3 fatty acids. Animal research shows that omega-3-deficient diets negatively affect the sleep hormone melatonin and its function and throw off the natural sleep cycle (our circadian rhythm), which can lead to sleep disturbances. Eating salmon and other fish rich in omega-3s is a good start to bolster proper levels.

Pumpkin Seeds

Low magnesium levels have been associated with inflammatory or oxidative stress and other factors that can interfere with a good night's sleep. Pumpkin seeds are rich in magnesium and also contain the amino acid tryptophan. A study on a close relative of the pumpkin seed found that the seeds were as effective in improving tryptophan levels as tryptophan supplements. Read more about pumpkin seeds' other benefits on page 83.

Lettuce

The natural oil that occurs in lettuce has been used in folk medicine as an aid to relaxation and for inducing sleep. A randomized, placebo-controlled study found that those given lettuce oil had markedly better sleep rating scores compared to the control group. Eating simply the lettuce itself (especially nutritious romaine; see page 189) may help you lull off.

Milk

A glass of warm milk has long been a folk remedy to promote a good night's sleep. Although the scientific literature is a bit thin on backing this up, the nutrients in milk, specifically calcium and tryptophan, are known to induce sleep. Calcium helps the brain use the amino acid tryptophan, and tryptophan is used to manufacture melatonin. Also, the carbohydrate in milk helps tryptophan work well, too! Turn to page 222 for more about milk.

Walnuts

Walnuts contain a number of nutrients that support a relaxed and healthy nervous system, including folate, melatonin, omega-3 fats, and vitamin E (see page 239 for the full lineup of this nut's healthy benefits). Research shows that the melatonin in walnuts is well absorbed and will raise blood melatonin concentrations when eaten in moderation, which in turn will help you get those zzzz's.

The Best Things You Can Eat, by Food/Beverage

Following, a food and beverage breakdown of the nutrients in the best things you can eat. Boldface indicates that the item is an excellent source of that nutrient; the item is a good source of nonbold nutrients.

Rankings and further discussion of all items in this table, and of the health benefits of all listed nutrients, can be found in Chapters 1 through 10.

Food	Excellent/Good Source of . . .
Acorn (winter) squash	**Fiber, iron, magnesium, manganese**, niacin, pantothenic acid, phosphorus, potassium, **thiamine, vitamin B$_6$, vitamin C**
Almonds	Copper, fiber, **vitamin E, manganese, magnesium**, phosphorus, protein
Amaranth	Copper, fiber, iron, **magnesium, manganese, phosphorus**, vitamin B$_6$
Apples	**Fiber**
Apricots	Fiber, potassium, **vitamin A**, vitamin C
Asparagus	Fiber, **folate, iron**, niacin, phosphorus, riboflavin, **thiamine**, vitamin A, vitamin B$_6$, vitamin C, vitamin E, **vitamin K**, zinc

continues

continued

Food	Excellent/Good Source of . . .
Artichokes	Copper, **fiber**, **folate**, niacin, magnesium, manganese, phosphorus, potassium, vitamin C, vitamin K
Avocados	**Monounsaturates**
Bananas	Fiber, manganese, potassium, **vitamin B$_6$**, vitamin C
Barley	Copper, **fiber**, magnesium, **manganese**, niacin, phosphorus, **selenium**, **thiamine**
Beans, black	**Fiber**, **folate**, **iron**, **magnesium**, **manganese**, **molybdenum**, **phosphorus**, potassium, **protein**, **thiamine**, zinc
Beans, kidney	**Fiber**, **folate**, **iron**, magnesium, **manganese**, **molybdenum**, **phosphorus**, **potassium**, **protein**, thiamine, vitamin K
Beans, lima	**Copper**, **fiber**, folate, **iron**, **magnesium**, **manganese**, **molybdenum**, **potassium**, **protein**, thiamine
Beans, pinto	**Fiber**, **folate**, **iron**, **manganese**, **molybdenum**, **phosphorus**, **protein**, thiamine
Beans, white/navy	Calcium, **fiber**, **folate**, **iron**, **magnesium**, **molybdenum**, **phosphorus**, **potassium**, **protein**, zinc
Beef	**Choline**, **chromium**, iron, niacin, **protein**, riboflavin, **selenium**, vitamin B$_6$, **zinc**
Beef liver	**Biotin**, **choline**, **chromium**, **copper**, **folate**, iron, **niacin**, **pantothenic acid**, **phosphorus**, **protein**, **riboflavin**, selenium, **vitamin A**, **vitamin B$_6$**, **vitamin B$_{12}$**, zinc
Beef, veal	**Choline**, **niacin**, **protein**, riboflavin, vitamin B$_{12}$, **zinc**
Beer	Chromium
Blueberries	Fiber, **manganese**, **vitamin C**, **vitamin K**
Brazil nuts	**Copper**, fiber, **magnesium**, manganese, **phosphorus**, **selenium**, thiamine
Brewer's yeast	**Chromium**, copper, **fiber**, **folic acid**, **iron**, **niacin**, **phosphorus**, **protein**, **riboflavin**, **selenium**, **thiamine**, **vitamin B$_6$**, **zinc**
Broccoli	**Chromium**, vitamin A, **vitamin C**, vitamin K
Buckwheat	**Choline**, magnesium
Canola oil	**Monounsaturates**, **omega-3 fats**, phytosterols, **vitamin E**
Carob powder	Fiber

continues

continued

Food	Excellent/Good Source of . . .
Carrots/carrot juice	**Alpha-carotene, beta-carotene,** lutein, **vitamin A,** zeaxanthin
Cheese, cottage	Calcium, **phosphorus, riboflavin,** vitamin B$_6$, **vitamin B$_{12}$**
Cheese, ricotta	**Calcium, phosphorus, protein, riboflavin,** vitamin A
Cheese, Parmesan/hard	**Calcium, chromium,** phosphorus, **protein**
Cherries	Fiber, vitamin C
Chia seeds	Calcium, **copper, iron,** magnesium, **manganese,** niacin, **omega-3 fats, phosphorus, selenium,** thiamine, **zinc**
Chicken	Choline, **niacin,** pantothenic acid, **protein,** selenium
Chicken liver	**Biotin, choline, folate, iron,** lutein, lycopene, **niacin, pantothenic acid, phosphorus, riboflavin, vitamin A, vitamin B$_{12}$,** zeaxanthin, **zinc**
Chicken soup	Iron, **sodium,** vitamin A
Chickpeas (garbanzo beans)	**Copper, fiber, folate,** magnesium, **manganese, molybdenum, protein, vitamin B$_6$**
Clams	Copper, **iron, manganese,** phosphorus, **potassium,** protein, riboflavin, **selenium, sodium, vitamin B$_{12}$,** vitamin C
Cocoa/cacao/chocolate	Copper
Cod/cod liver oil	**Iodine, magnesium, niacin,** omega-3 fatty acids (oil), **phosphorus, selenium, sodium, vitamin A** (oil), **vitamin B$_6$, vitamin B$_{12}$, vitamin D** (oil), **vitamin E** (oil)
Coffee	Coffee is not a significant source of any one nutrient; however it does supply important phytochemicals, such as polyphenols.
Corn	Fiber, manganese, niacin, **pantothenic acid,** vitamin C
Corn oil	Phytosterols, **polyunsaturates**
Cowpeas (black-eyed peas)	**Biotin, calcium, fiber, folate,** iron, **magnesium, manganese, molybdenum,** niacin, potassium, **protein,** thiamine, vitamin A, **vitamin K,** zinc
Crab	**Copper,** magnesium, niacin, phosphorus, **protein,** riboflavin, **sodium, vitamin B$_{12}$,** vitamin C, **zinc**
Cranberries	Fiber, vitamin C
Eggs	**Biotin, choline, iodine,** phosphorus, **protein,** riboflavin, vitamin D

continues

continued

Food	Excellent/Good Source of . . .
Elderberries	**Vitamin A**, vitamin C
Figs	Calcium, **fiber**, iron, **magnesium**, **manganese**, pantothenic acid, phosphorus, thiamine, vitamin B$_6$
Flaxseeds/flaxseed oil	Fiber (seeds), magnesium (seeds), **omega-3 fats**, phosphorus (seeds), **polyunsaturates**
Garlic	Garlic is not a significant source of any one nutrient, but contains important phytochemicals such as alliin, allicin, and saponins.
Ginger	Ginger is not a significant source of any one nutrient, but contains important phytonutrients such as gingerols, shogaols, and zingerones.
Grapes/grape juice	**Chromium, manganese, vitamin C**
Grapeseed oil	**Polyunsaturates, vitamin E**
Greens, beet	**Potassium**, riboflavin, **sodium**, **vitamin A**, **vitamin C**, **vitamin K**
Greens, collard	**Calcium**, fiber, **folate**, iron, **manganese**, **vitamin A**, **vitamin C**, **vitamin K**
Greens, dandelion	Calcium, **vitamin A, vitamin C, vitamin K**
Greens, turnip	Copper, fiber, **folate**, **manganese**, **vitamin A**, vitamin B$_6$, **vitamin C**, vitamin E, **vitamin K**
Guavas	**Fiber, folate, lycopene**, potassium, **vitamin A, vitamin C**
Halibut	**Magnesium, niacin**, omega-3 fats, **phosphorus, protein, selenium**, vitamin B$_{12}$
Hazelnuts (filberts)	**Copper, fiber, magnesium, manganese, monounsaturates, vitamin E**
Herring	**Monounsaturates, niacin, omega-3 fats, phosphorus, protein, riboflavin, selenium, vitamin B$_6$, vitamin B$_{12}$**
Honey	Honey is not significant source of any one nutrient, but darker varieties contain important antioxidants.
Jerusalem artichokes	**Fiber, iron**, vitamin C
Kale	Calcium, fiber, iron, phosphorus, **vitamin A**, vitamin B$_6$, **vitamin C, vitamin K**
Kamut	Calcium, **copper**, **fiber**, **iron**, **magnesium**, **manganese**, **phosphorus**, **potassium**, protein, **thiamine**, vitamin E, **zinc**

continues

continued

Food	Excellent/Good Source of . . .
Kefir	**Calcium**, folate, magnesium, protein, riboflavin, vitamin B$_{12}$
Kiwis	**Fiber**, folate, potassium, **vitamin C**
Lamb	**Choline**, iron, **pantothenic acid**, phosphorus, **protein**, **selenium, vitamin B$_{12}$, zinc**
Lentils	**Biotin, fiber, folate**, iron, **magnesium, manganese, molybdenum, phosphorus, potassium, thiamine, vitamin B$_6$, zinc**
Lettuce, romaine	**Vitamin A, vitamin C**
Lobster	**Copper, pantothenic acid**, phosphorus, **protein**, selenium, **sodium, zinc**
Macadamia nuts	Fiber, **manganese, monounsaturates**, thiamine
Milk	**Calcium, iodine, phosphorus, riboflavin**, vitamin A, **vitamin B$_{12}$, vitamin D**, zinc
Millet	Choline
Mushrooms, shiitake	**Copper**, niacin, **pantothenic acid**, phosphorus, riboflavin, vitamin B$_6$, **vitamin D**
Mushrooms, white/portobello	**Biotin, copper, chromium, niacin**, pantothenic acid, **riboflavin, selenium**, vitamin D
Oats	Fiber, phosphorus
Okra	Calcium, folate, fiber, magnesium, vitamin B$_6$, **vitamin C, vitamin K**
Olives/olive oil (extra-virgin)	**Monounsaturates**, vitamin E
Onions	**Vitamin K**
Oranges/orange juice	Folate, potassium, **Vitamin C**
Orange roughy	**Protein, selenium**
Oysters	**Copper, iron**, magnesium, phosphorus, **protein**, riboflavin, **selenium, vitamin B$_{12}$, zinc**
Papayas	Fiber, folate, **vitamin A, vitamin C**
Peanuts/peanut butter	**Biotin**, fiber, folate, magnesium, **manganese**, niacin, phosphorus, protein, riboflavin, sodium, vitamin E
Pears	**Fiber**, vitamin C
Peas, green	**Fiber, folate**, iron, **lutein**, magnesium, niacin, phosphorus, potassium, **protein, vitamin A, vitamin C, vitamin K, zeaxanthin**

continues

continued

Food	Excellent/Good Source of . . .
Peas, yellow split	Choline, **fiber**, **folate**, **iron**, magnesium, **manganese**, **molybdenum**, niacin, **pantothenic acid**, **phosphorus**, potassium, **thiamine**, zinc
Pecans	Fiber, **monounsaturates**
Peppermint	Peppermint is not a significant source of any one nutrient, but contains important phytonutrients, such as menthol, limonene, eucalyptol, and pinene.
Peppers	Folate, lycopene, **vitamin A**, **vitamin C**
Pineapple	**Manganese**, **vitamin C**
Pine nuts	Copper, iron, **manganese**, magnesium, **polyunsaturates**, zinc
Pistachios	**Copper**, **manganese**, phosphorus, phytosterols
Plums, dried (prunes)	Fiber, vitamin A, **vitamin B$_6$**
Pork	**Biotin**, **choline**, **niacin**, **protein**, **selenium**, **thiamine**, **vitamin B$_6$**, **vitamin B$_{12}$**, zinc
Pork sausage (braunschweiger)	**Choline**, iron, niacin, **pantothenic acid**, **protein**, selenium, **vitamin A**, **vitamin B$_{12}$**
Potatoes	**Potassium**, vitamin B$_6$, **vitamin C**
Psyllium husks	**Fiber**
Pumpkin/pumpkin seeds	**Fiber**, **copper** (seeds), iron (seeds), **magnesium** (seeds), **manganese** (seeds), **phosphorus** (seeds), **vitamin A**, zinc (seeds)
Quinoa	Copper, fiber, **folic acid**, iron, **magnesium**, **manganese**, **phosphorus**, protein, thiamine, vitamin B$_6$
Raisins	Raisins are not a significant source of any one nutrient, but are a source of important phytonutrients, such as quinic and gallic acid, chlorogenic and caffeic acids, catechin, and epicatechins.
Raspberries	**Fiber**, **manganese**, **vitamin C**, vitamin K
Rice	Magnesium, selenium
Rice bran oil	Phytosterols, **vitamin E**
Rhubarb	**Calcium**, **fiber**
Rockfish	**Choline**, potassium, **selenium**
Sablefish	Iron, magnesium, **niacin**, **omega-3 fats**, **phosphorus**, **potassium**, **protein**, **selenium**, **vitamin B$_6$**, **vitamin B$_{12}$**

continues

continued

Food	Excellent/Good Source of . . .
Safflower oil	**Monounsaturates, vitamin E**
Salmon	**Biotin, choline, niacin, omega-3 fats**, pantothenic acid, phosphorus, **potassium, protein, selenium, vitamin B$_6$, vitamin B$_{12}$**
Salt, iodized	**Iodine, sodium**
Sapodillas	Copper, **fiber**, folate, iron, niacin, pantothenic acid, potassium, **vitamin A, vitamin C**
Sardines	**Calcium, niacin, omega-3 fats, phosphorus, protein, vitamin B$_{12}$**
Seaweed (kombu)	**Iodine, sodium**
Sesame seeds/sesame oil	**Calcium, copper, iron, magnesium, manganese**, phosphorus, phytosterols, thiamine, vitamin B$_6$, zinc
Shrimp	Copper, **iodine**, niacin, **phosphorus, protein, selenium**, vitamin B$_6$, **vitamin B$_{12}$**, zinc.
Sorghum	Sorghum is not a significant source of any one nutrient, but contains important phytochemicals, such as flavonoids and proanthocyanins.
Soy	**Calcium, fiber, folate, iron, magnesium**, niacin, **omega-3 fats, phosphorus, polyunsaturates, potassium, protein, riboflavin, thiamine**, vitamin C, **vitamin K**, zinc
Spinach	**Calcium**, fiber, **folate, iron, magnesium, manganese**, phosphorus, **potassium, riboflavin**, thiamine, **vitamin A, vitamin B$_6$, vitamin C, vitamin E, vitamin K**, zinc
Strawberries	Anthocyanins, catechins, ellagic acid, flavonoids, folate, **vitamin C**
Sunflower seeds/sunflower oil	**Copper**, fiber, folate, **magnesium**, phosphorus, phytosterols, **polyunsaturates**, protein, **selenium, vitamin E**
Sweet potatoes	**Fiber**, iron, magnesium, niacin, phosphorus, **potassium**, riboflavin, thiamine, **vitamin A, vitamin B$_6$, vitamin C**
Swiss chard	Calcium, fiber, **iron, magnesium, potassium, sodium, vitamin A, vitamin C, vitamin K**
Swordfish	Choline, **omega-3 fats, protein, selenium**, vitamin B$_6$, vitamin B$_{12}$
Tea, black	Black tea is not a significant source of any one nutrient, but does contain important phytonutrients, such as flavonols.

continues

continued

Food	Excellent/Good Source of . . .
Tea, green	Green tea is not a significant source of any one nutrient, but contains important phytochemicals, such as epicatechins.
Teff	**Copper**, fiber, iron, magnesium, **manganese**, phosphorus, protein, thiamine, vitamin B$_6$, zinc
Tomatoes	Potassium, **vitamin A**, **vitamin C**, vitamin K
Triticale	Copper, **fiber**, magnesium, **manganese**, niacin, phosphorus, protein, thiamine, zinc
Trout, rainbow	Niacin, **omega-3 fats, pantothenic acid, protein**, selenium
Tuna, yellowfin	**Niacin**, omega-3 fats, pantothenic acid, **protein**, selenium, vitamin B$_6$, vitamin B$_{12}$
Turkey	Iron, **protein**, riboflavin, thiamine, vitamin B$_6$, vitamin B$_{12}$, **zinc**
Turkey giblets	**Iron, folate, niacin, phosphorus, protein, riboflavin, vitamin A, vitamin B$_{12}$, zinc**
Turmeric	Turmeric is not a significant source of any one nutrient, but does contain important phytonutrients, such as curcumin.
Walleye	Choline, niacin, **phosphorus**, potassium, **protein, selenium, sodium**, vitamin B$_{12}$
Walnuts	**Copper**, iron, magnesium, **manganese, omega-3 fats**, phosphorus, **polyunsaturates, vitamin E**
Watermelon	**Magnesium** (seeds), **phosphorus** (seeds), **vitamin A, vitamin C**, zinc (seeds)
Wheat/bulgur	Copper, **fiber**, magnesium, **manganese**, niacin, **phosphorus**, protein, **selenium**, thiamine, vitamin B$_6$
Wheat bran	**Fiber, phosphorus**
Wheat germ oil	**Vitamin E**
Whey	**Calcium, protein**
Wine	**Chromium**
Yeast, brewer's	**B-complex vitamins, chromium, protein, selenium, vitamin B$_{12}$**
Yogurt	**Calcium, iodine, pantothenic acid, phosphorus, potassium, protein, riboflavin, vitamin B$_{12}$**

Bibliography

CHAPTER 1: THE VITA-MAN CAN

Billing, J. and P. W. Sherman. "Antimicrobial Functions of Spices: Why Some Like It Hot." *Quarterly Review of Biology* 73, no. 1 (March 1998): 3–49.

Bondonno, C. P., et al. "Flavonoid-Rich Apples and Nitrate-Rich Spinach Augment Nitric Oxide Status and Improve Endothelial Function in Healthy Men and Women: A Randomized Controlled Trial." *Free Radical Biology and Medicine* 52, no. 1 (January 1, 2012): 95–102.

Cockayne, S., et al. "Vitamin K and the Prevention of Fractures: Systematic Review and Meta-analysis of Randomized Controlled Trials." *Archives of International Medicine* 166, no. 12 (2006): 1256–61.

Denter, J., and B. Bisping. "Formation of B-vitamins by Bacteria During the Soaking Process of Soybeans for Tempe Fermentation." *International Journal of Food Microbiology* 22, no. 1 (April 1994): 23–31.

Deyhim, F., et al. "Orange Pulp Improves Antioxidant Status and Suppresses Lipid Peroxidation in Orchidectomized Male Rats." *Nutrition* 23, no. 7–8 (July–August 2007): 617–21.

Dietary Supplement Fact Sheet: Vitamin B_{12}. Retrieved from http://ods.od.nih .gov/factsheets/vitaminb12 on March 3, 2012.

Esmaillzadeh, A., and L. Azadbakht. "Legume Consumption Is Inversely Associated with Serum Concentrations of Adhesion Molecules and Inflammatory Biomarkers Among Iranian Women." *Journal of Nutrition* 142, no. 2 (February 2012): 334–39.

Eussen, S. J., et al. "Plasma Vitamins B_2, B_6, and B_{12}, and Related Genetic Variants as Predictors of Colorectal Cancer Risk." *Cancer Epidemiology Biomarkers & Prevention* 19, no. 10 (October 2010): 2549–61.

García-Rodríguez, C. E., et al. "Does Consumption of Two Portions of Salmon per Week Enhance the Antioxidant Defense System in Pregnant Women?" *Antioxidants & Redox Signaling* 16, no. 12 (June 15, 2012): 1401–6.

Kim, S. Y., et al. "Kale Juice Improves Coronary Artery Disease Risk Factors in Hypercholesterolemic Men." *Biomedical and Environmental Sciences* 21, no. 2 (April 2008): 91–97.

Klein, E. A., et al. "Vitamin E and the Risk of Prostate Cancer: The Selenium and Vitamin E Cancer Prevention Trial (SELECT)." *Journal of the American Medical Association* 306, no. 14 (October 12, 2011): 1549–56.

Kobayashi, D., et al. "The Effect of Pantothenic Acid Deficiency on Keratinocyte Proliferation and the Synthesis of Keratinocyte Growth Factor and Collagen in Fibroblasts." *Journal of Pharmacological Sciences* 115, no. 2 (2011): 230–34.

Krinsky N. I., J. T. Landrum, and R. A. Bone. "Biologic Mechanisms of the Protective Role of Lutein and Zeaxanthin in the Eye." *Annual Review of Nutrition* 23 (2003): 171–201.

McGowan, C. A., et al. "Insufficient Vitamin D Intakes Among Pregnant Women." *European Journal of Clinical Nutrition* 65, no. 9 (September 2011): 1076–78.

Mousain-Bosc, M., et al. "Improvement of Neurobehavioral Disorders in Children Supplemented with Magnesium–Vitamin B_6. II. Pervasive Developmental Disorder-Autism." *Magnesium Research* 19, no. 1 (March 2006): 53–62.

Murakoshi, M., et al. "Potent Preventive Action of Alpha-Carotene Against Carcinogenesis: Spontaneous Liver Carcinogenesis and Promoting Stage of Lung and Skin Carcinogenesis in Mice Are Suppressed More Effectively by Alpha-Carotene than by Beta-Carotene." *Cancer Research* 52, no. 23 (December 1, 1992): 6583–87.

Murphy, M. M., et al. "Fresh and Fresh Lean Pork Are Substantial Sources of Key Nutrients When These Products Are Consumed by Adults in the United States." *Nutrition Research* 31, no. 10 (October 2011): 776–83.

Naghashpour, M., et al. "Riboflavin Status and Its Association with Serum hs-CRP Levels Among Clinical Nurses with Depression." *Journal of the American College of Nutrition* 30, no. 5 (October 2011): 340–47.

Pelletier, S. X., et al. "A Diet Moderately Enriched in Phytosterols Lowers Plasma Cholesterol Concentrations in Normocholesterolemic Humans." *Annals of Nutrition and Metabolism* 39 (1995): 291–95.

Praxedes de Aquino, R. C., et al. "Analysis of Retinol Concentrations in Bovine Liver and Its Habitual Consumption by Pregnant Women." *Annals of Nutrition and Metabolism* 50, no. 4 (2006): 325–29.

Rabbani, R., et al. "High-Dose Thiamine Therapy for Patients with Type 2 Diabetes and Microalbuminuria: A Randomised, Double-Blind Placebo-Controlled Pilot Study." *Diabetologia* 52, no. 2 (February 2009): 208–12.

Reis, F. S., et al. "Composition and Nutritional Value of the Most Widely Appreciated Cultivated Mushrooms: An Inter-species Comparative Study." *Food and Chemical Toxicology* (October 28, 2011).

Schaefer, E. J., et al. "Plasma Phosphatidylcholine Docosahexaenoic Acid Content and Risk of Dementia and Alzheimer Disease: The Framingham Heart Study." *Archives of Neurology* 63, no. 11 (November 2006): 1545–50.

Sconce, E., P. Avery, P. Wynne, and F. Kamali. "Vitamin K Supplementation Can Improve Stability of Anticoagulation for Patients with Unexplained Variability in Response to Warfarin." *Blood* 109, no. 6 (2007): 2419–23.

Ueta, Kazumi, et al. "Broth from Canned Clams Is Suitable for Use as an Excellent Source of Free Vitamin B_{12}." *Journal of Agricultural and Food Chemistry* 59, no. 22 (2011): 12054–58. Retrieved from http://pubs.acs.org/doi/abs/10.1021/jf2037104 on February 20, 2012.

Yong, L. C., and M. R. Petersen. "High Dietary Niacin Intake Is Associated with Decreased Chromosome Translocation Frequency in Airline Pilots." *British Journal of Nutrition* 105, no. 4 (February 2011): 496–505.

Yu, B. H., and C. Kies. "Niacin, Thiamine, and Pantothenic Acid Bioavailability to Humans from Maize Bran as Affected by Milling and Particle Size." *Plant Foods for Human Nutrition* 43, no. 1 (January 1993): 87–95.

Zhang, R., and D. P. Naughton. "Vitamin D in Health and Disease: Current Perspectives." *Nutrition Journal* 9, no. 65 (2010).

CHAPTER 2: DIGGING THE MINERALS

Adams, L. S., et al. "White Button Mushroom (*Agaricus bisporus*) Exhibits Antiproliferative and Proapoptotic Properties and Inhibits Prostate Tumor Growth in Athymic Mice." *Nutrition and Cancer* 60, no. 6 (2008): 744–56.

Berr, C., et al. "Increased Selenium Intake in Elderly High Fish Consumers May Account for Health Benefits Previously Ascribed to Omega-3 Fatty Acids." *Journal of Nutrition Health & Aging* 13, no. 1 (January 2009): 14–18.

Centers for Disease Control and Prevention (CDC). "CDC Grand Rounds: Dietary Sodium Reduction—Time for Choice." MMWR Morbidity and Mortality Weekly Report February 10, 2012. 61(05); 89–91. http://www.cdc.gov/salt/pdfs/sodium_fact_sheet.pdf accessed March 29, 2012.

Freedman, M. R., and D. R. Keast. "White Potatoes, Including French Fries, Contribute Shortfall Nutrients to Children's and Adolescents' Diets." *Nutrition Research* 31, no. 4 (April 2011): 270–77.

Fulgoni, V. L. III, et al. "Nutrients from Dairy Foods Are Difficult to Replace in Diets of Americans: Food Pattern Modeling and an Analysis of the National Health And Nutrition Examination Survey 2003–2006." *Nutrition Research* 31, no. 10 (October 2011): 759–65.

Gennari, C. "Calcium and Vitamin D Nutrition and Bone Disease of the Elderly." *Public Health Nutrition* 4, no. 2B (April 2001): 547–59.

Gletsu-Miller, N., et al. "Incidence and Prevalence of Copper Deficiency Following Roux-en-y Gastric Bypass Surgery." *International Journal of Obesity* 36, no. 3 (March 2012): 328–35.

Grimm, M., et al. "High Phosphorus Intake Only Slightly Affects Serum Minerals, Urinary Pyridinium Crosslinks and Renal Function in Young Women." *European Journal of Clinical Nutrition* 55, no. 3 (2001): 153–61.

Hale, L. P., et al. "Dietary Supplementation with Fresh Pineapple Juice Decreases Inflammation and Colonic Neoplasia in IL-10-Deficient Mice with Colitis." *Inflammatory Bowel Diseases* 16, no. 12 (December 2010): 2012–21.

Hu, Y., et al. "Kaempferol in Red and Pinto Bean Seed (*Phaseolus vulgaris L.*) Coats Inhibits Iron Bioavailability Using an in Vitro Digestion/Human Caco-2 Cell Model." *Journal of Agricultural and Food Chemistry* 54, no. 24 (November 29, 2006): 9254–61.

Josse, A. R., et al. "Almonds and Postprandial Glycemia—A Dose-Response Study." *Metabolism* 56, no. 3 (March 2007): 400–404.

Karp, H., et al. "Differences Among Total and in Vitro Digestible Phosphorus Content of Meat and Milk Products." *Journal of Renal Nutrition* 22, no. 3 (May 2012): 344–49.

Khosravi-Boroujeni, H., et al. "Favorable Effects on Metabolic Risk Factors with Daily Brewer's Yeast in Type 2 Diabetic Patients with Hypercholesterolemia: A Semi-Experimental Study." *Journal of Diabetes* 4, no. 2 (June 2012): 153–58.

Kristensen, M. B., et al. "Total Zinc Absorption in Young Women, but Not Fractional Zinc Absorption, Differs Between Vegetarian and Meat-Based Diets with Equal Phytic Acid Content." *British Journal of Nutrition* 95, no. 5 (May 2006): 963–67.

Marlett, J. A., M. I. McBurney, and J. L. Slavin. "Position of the American Dietetic Association: Health Implications of Dietary Fiber." *Journal of the American Dietetic Association* 102, no. 7 (July 2002): 993–1000.

Mitchell, D. C., et al. "Consumption of Dry Beans, Peas, and Lentils Could Improve Diet Quality in the U.S. Population." *Journal of the American Dietetic Association* 109, no. 5 (May 2009): 909–13.

O'Neil, C. E., et al. "Tree Nut Consumption Improves Nutrient Intake and Diet Quality in U.S. Adults: An Analysis of National Health and Nutrition Examination Survey (NHANES) 1999–2004." *Asia Pacific Journal of Clinical Nutrition* 19, no. 1 (2010): 142–50.

Pearce, E. N. "National Trends in Iodine Nutrition: Is Everyone Getting Enough?" *Thyroid* 17, no. 8 (September 2007): 823–27.

Pearce, E. N., et al. "Sources of Dietary Iodine: Bread, Cows' Milk, and Infant Formula in the Boston Area." *Journal of Clinical Endocrinology & Metabolism* 89, no. 7 (July 2004): 3421–24.

Rao, A. V., and D. M. Snyder. "Raspberries and Human Health: A Review." *Journal of Agricultural and Food Chemistry* 58, no. 7 (April 14, 2010): 3871–83.

Rude, R. K. "Magnesium Deficiency: A Cause of Heterogeneous Disease in Humans." *Journal of Bone and Mineral Research* 12 (1993): 749–58.

Saris, N. E., et al. "Magnesium: An Update on Physiological, Clinical, and Analytical Aspects." *Clinica Chimica Acta* 294 (2000): 1–26.

Singh, M., and R. R. Das. "Zinc for the Common Cold." Cochrane Database of Systematic Reviews (February 16, 2011): 2:CD001364.

Stranges, S., et al. "A Prospective Study of Dietary Selenium Intake and Risk of Type 2 Diabetes." *BMC Public Health* 10 (September 21, 2010): 564.

Tordoff, M. G., and M. A. Sandell. "Vegetable Bitterness Is Related to Calcium Content." *Appetite* 52, no. 2 (April 2009): 498–504.

CHAPTER 3: CHEWING THE FATS, FIBER, AND PHYTOSTEROLS

Agurs-Collins, T., et al. "Legume Intake and Reduced Colorectal Adenoma Risk in African-Americans." *Journal of National Black Nurses Association* 17, no. 2 (December 2006): 6–12.

Asp, M. L., et al. "Time-Dependent Effects of Safflower Oil to Improve Glycemia, Inflammation and Blood Lipids in Obese, Post-Menopausal Women with Type 2 Diabetes: A Randomized, Double-Masked, Crossover Study." *Clinical Nutrition* 30, no. 4 (August 2011): 443–49.

Bassett, C. M., et al. "The α-linolenic Acid Content of Flaxseed Can Prevent the Atherogenic Effects of Dietary Trans Fat." *American Journal of Physiology—Heart and Circulatory Physiology* 301, no. 6 (December 2011): H2220–26.

Cyril, W. C., et al. "Nuts, Metabolic Syndrome and Diabetes." *British Journal of Nutrition* 104 (2010): 465–73.

Gouni-Berthold, I., and H. K. Berthold. "Policosanol: Clinical Pharmacology and Therapeutic Significance of New Lipid-Lowering Agent." *American Heart Journal* 143, no. 2 (2002): 356–65.

Griel, A. E., et al. "A Macadamia Nut–Rich Diet Reduces Total and LDL-Cholesterol in Mildly Hypercholesterolemic Men and Women." *Journal of Nutrition* 138, no. 4 (April 2008): 761–67.

Harris, W. S., et al. "Omega-6 Fatty Acids and Risk for Cardiovascular Disease: A Science Advisory from the American Heart Association Nutrition Subcommittee of the Council on Nutrition, Physical Activity, and Metabolism; Council on Cardiovascular Nursing; and Council on Epidemiology and Prevention." *Circulation* 119 (2009): 902–7.

Heber, D., and S. Bowerman. "Applying Science to Changing Dietary Patterns." *Journal of Nutrition* 131, no. 11 (November 2001): 3078S–81S.

Murty, C. M., et al. "Chickpea Supplementation in an Australian Diet Affects Food Choice, Satiety and Bowel Health." *Appetite* 54, no. 2 (April 2010): 282–88.

Musa-Veloso, K., et al. "A Comparison of the LDL-Cholesterol Lowering Efficacy of Plant Stanols and Plant Sterols over a Continuous Dose Range: Results of a Meta-Analysis of Randomized, Placebo-Controlled Trials." *Prostaglandins Leukotrienes and Essential Fatty Acids* 85, no. 1 (July 2011): 9–28.

Ulbricht, C., et al. "Chia (*Salvia hispanica*): A Systematic Review by the Natural Standard Research Collaboration." *Reviews on Recent Clinical Trials* 4 (2009): 168–74.

Wong, J. M., et al. "The Effect on the Blood Lipid Profile of Soy Foods Combined with a Prebiotic: A Randomized Controlled Trial." *Metabolism* 59, no. 2 (September 2010): 1331–40.

CHAPTER 4: DIGEST THIS!

Chen, S., J. Wang, and Y. Li. "Is Alcohol Consumption Associated with Gastro-esophageal Reflux Disease?" *Journal of Zhejiang University* 11, no. 6 (June 2010): 423–28.

Hargrove, J. L., et al. "Inhibition of Aromatase and α-amylase by Flavonoids and Proanthocyanidins from Sorghum Bicolor Bran Extracts." *Journal of Medicinal Food* 14, no. 7–8 (July–August 2011): 799–807.

Li, S. Q., and Q. H. Zhang. "Advances in the Development of Functional Foods from Buckwheat." *Critical Reviews in Food Science and Nutrition* 41, no. 6 (September 2001): 451–64.

Loeb, H., et al. "Tannin-Rich Carob Pod for the Treatment of Acute-Onset Diarrhea." *Journal of Pediatric Gastroenterology and Nutrition* 8, no. 4 (1989): 480–85.

McFarland, L. V. "Evidence-Based Review of Probiotics for Antibiotic-Associated Diarrhea and *Clostridium difficile* Infections." *Anaerobe* 15, no. 6 (2009): 274–80.

Trinkley, K. E., K. Porter, and M. C. Nahata. "Prescribing Patterns for the Outpatient Treatment of Constipation in the United States." *Digestive Diseases and Sciences* 55, no. 12 (December 2010): 3514–20.

CHAPTER 5: HEARTY FOODS

Cesar, T. B., et al. "Orange Juice Decreases Low-Density Lipoprotein Cholesterol in Hypercholesterolemic Subjects and Improves Lipid Transfer to High-Density Lipoprotein in Normal and Hypercholesterolemic Subjects." *Nutrition Research* 30, no. 10 (October 2010): 689–94.

Estévez-González. M. D., et al. "HDL Cholesterol Levels in Children with Mild Hypercholesterolemia: Effect of Consuming Skim Milk Enriched with Olive Oil and Modulation by the TAQ 1B Polymorphism in the CETP Gene." *Annals of Nutrition and Metabolism* 56, no. 4 (2010): 288–93.

Inoue, N., et al. "Screening of Soy Protein-Derived Hypotriglyceridemic Di-peptides in Vitro and in Vivo." *Lipids in Health and Disease* 10 (May 22, 2011): 85.

Jalali-Khanabadi, B. A., et al. "Effects of Almond Dietary Supplementation on Coronary Heart Disease Lipid Risk Factors and Serum Lipid Oxidation Parameters in Men with Mild Hyperlipidemia." *Journal of Alternative and Complementary Medicine* 16, no. 12 (December): 1279–83.

Rasmussen, B., E. Vessby, and M. Uusitupa. "Effects of Dietary Saturated, Monounsaturated, and n-3 Fatty Acids on Blood Pressure in Healthy Subjects." *American Journal of Clinical Nutrition* 83, no. 2 (February 2006): 221–26.

Shearer, G. C., C. V. Savinova, and W. S. Harris. "Fish Oil: How Does It Reduce Plasma Triglycerides?" *Biochimica et Biophysica Acta* 1821, no. 5 (May 2012): 843–51.

Yang, S. C., et al. "Soybean Protein Hydrolysate Improves Plasma and Liver Lipid Profiles in Rats Fed High-Cholesterol Diet." *Journal of the American College of Nutrition* 26 (2007): 416–23.

CHAPTER 6: SUGAR BLUES

Butt, M. S., et al. "Oat: Unique Among the Cereals." *European Journal of Nutrition* 47 (2008): 68–79.

Husband, A. C., et al. "The Effectiveness of Glucose, Sucrose, and Fructose in Treating Hypoglycemia in Children with Type 1 Diabetes." *Pediatric Diabetes* 11 (2010): 154–58.

Kim, H., et al. "Glucose and Insulin Responses to Whole Grain Breakfasts Varying in Soluble Fiber, Beta-glucan." *European Journal of Nutrition* 48 (2009): 170–75.

Rovner, A. J., et al. "The Effect of a Low-Glycemic Diet vs. a Standard Diet on Blood Glucose Levels and Macronutrient Intake in Children with Type 1 Diabetes." *Journal of the American Dietetic Association* 109 (2009): 2, 303–7.

CHAPTER 7: ORAL MAJORITY

Hansanugrum, A., et al. "Effect of Milk on the Deodorization of Malodorous Breath after Garlic Ingestion." *Journal of Food Science* 75, no. 6 (2010): C549–58.

Negishi, O., and Y. Negishi. "Enzymatic Deodorization with Raw Fruits, Vegetables and Mushrooms." *Food Science and Technology Research* 5, no. 2 (1999): 176–80.

Osawa, K., et al. "Identification of Cariostatic Substances in the Cacao Bean Husk: Their Anti-glucosyltransferase and Antibacterial Activities." *Journal of Dental Research* 80, no. 11 (November 2001): 2000–2004.

Tanaka, K., et al. "Intake of Dairy Products and the Prevalence of Dental Caries in Young Children." *Journal of Dentistry* 38, no. 7 (2010): 579–83.

Venkateswara, B., et al. "Green Tea Extract for Periodontal Health." *Journal of Indian Society for Periodontology* 15, no. 1 (2011): 18–22.

CHAPTER 8: BEST FOR INSIDE AND OUT

Black, C. D., et al. "Ginger (*Zingiber officinale*) Reduces Muscle Pain Caused by Eccentric Exercise." *Journal of Pain* 11, no. 9 (September 2010): 894–903.

Hunger, D. C., et al. "Consumption of Gold Kiwifruit Reduces Severity and Duration of Selected Upper Respiratory Tract Infection Symptoms and Increases Plasma Vitamin C Concentration in Healthy Older Adults." *British Journal of Nutrition* 15 (2011): 1–11.

Kirsh, V. A., et al., "Prospective Study of Fruit and Vegetable Intake and Risk of Prostate Cancer." *Journal of the National Cancer Institute* 99, no. 15 (2007): 1200–1209.

Ndiaye, M., et al. "The Grape Antioxidant Resveratrol for Skin Disorders: Promise, Prospects, and Challenges." *Archives of Biochemistry and Biophysics* 508, no. 2 (April 15, 2011): 164–70.

Rahbar, N., N. Asgharzadeh, and R. Ghorbani. "Effect of Omega-3 Fatty Acids on Intensity of Primary Dysmenorrhea." *International Journal of Gynaecology and Obstetrics* 117, no. 1 (April 2012): 45–47.

Tokuyama, S., and K. Nakamoto. "Unsaturated Fatty Acids and Pain." *Biological & Pharmaceutical Bulletin* 34, no. 8 (2011): 1174–78.

Uchide, N., and H. Toyoda. "Antioxidant Therapy as a Potential Approach to Severe Influenza-Associated Complications." *Molecules* 16, no. 3 (2011): 2032–52.

Williams, S., S. Tamburic, and C. Lally. "Eating Chocolate Can Significantly Protect the Skin from UV Light." *Journal of Cosmetic Dermatology* 8, no. 3 (September 2009): 69–73.

Zhang, M., et al. "Antioxidant Properties of Quercetin." *Advances in Experimental Medicine and Science* 701 (2011): 283–89.

CHAPTER 9:
FOOD CATEGORY SUPERSTARS

Agil, R., and F. Hosseinian. "Dual Functionality of Triticale as a Novel Dietary Source of Prebiotics with Antioxidant Activity in Fermented Dairy Products." *Plant Foods for Human Nutrition* 67, no. 1 (March 2012): 88–93.

Basu, J., A. Sachdeva, and J. Nagpal. "Emerging Health Properties of Fermented Milk and Whey Proteins: Role in *Helicobacter pylori* Eradication." *Journal of Clinical Gastroenterology* 43, no. 10 (November–December 2009): 1011–12.

Bolling, B. W., et al. "Tree Nut Phytochemicals: Composition, Antioxidant Capacity, Bioactivity, Impact Factors. A Systematic Review of Almonds, Brazils, Cashews. Hazelnuts, Macadamias, Pecans, Pine Nuts, Pistachios and Walnuts." *Nutrition Research Reviews* 24, no. 2 (December 2011): 244–75.

Brown, M. J., et al. "Carotenoid Bioavailability Is Higher from Salads Ingested with Full-Fat Than with Fat-Reduced Salad Dressings as Measured with Electrochemical Detection." *American Journal of Clinical Nutrition* 80, no. 2 (August 2004): 396–403.

Davidi, A., et al. "The Effect of the Addition of Daily Fruit and Nut Bars to Diet on Weight, and Cardiac Risk Profile, in Overweight Adults." *Journal of Human Nutrition and Dietetics* 24, no. 6 (December 2011): 543–51.

Dhandayuthapani, S., et al. "Bromelain-Induced Apoptosis in GI-101A Breast Cancer Cells." *Journal of Medicinal Food* 15, no. 4 (April 2012): 344–49.

Iwasawa, H., et al. "Anti-oxidant Effects of Kiwi Fruit in Vitro and in Vivo." *Biological & Pharmaceutical Bulletin* 34, no. 1 (2011): 128–34.

Jonnalagadda, S. S., et al. "Putting the Whole Grain Puzzle Together: Health Benefits Associated with Whole Grains—Summary of American Society for Nutrition 2010 Satellite Symposium." *Journal of Nutrition* 141, no. 5 (May 2011): 1011S–22S

Paddon-Jones, D., et al. "Role of Dietary Protein in the Sarcopenia of Aging." *American Journal of Clinical Nutrition* 87 (2008): 1562S–66S.

Pelchat, M. L., et al. "Excretion and Perception of a Characteristic Odor in Urine After Asparagus Ingestion: A Psychophysical and Genetic Study." *Chemical Senses* 36, no. 1 (January 2011): 9–17.

Slatnar, A., et al. "Effect of Drying of Figs (*Ficus carica* L.) on the Contents of Sugars, Organic Acids, and Phenolic Compounds." *Journal of Agricultural and Food Chemistry* 59, no. 21 (November 9, 2011): 11696–1702.

Spaccarotella, K. J., and W. D. Andzel. "The Effects of Low Fat Chocolate Milk on Postexercise Recovery in Collegiate Athletes." *Journal of Strength and Conditioning Research* 25, no. 12 (December 2011): 3456–60.

Symons, T., et al. "Aging Does Not Impair the Anabolic Response to a Protein-Rich Meal." *American Journal of Clinical Nutrition* 86 (2007): 451–56.

Van Camp, D, N. H. Hooker, and C. T. Lin. "Changes in Fat Contents of U.S. Snack Foods in Response to Mandatory Trans Fat Labelling." *Public Health Nutrition* (February 8, 2012): 1–8.

Waller, S. M., et al. "Evening Ready-to-Eat Cereal Consumption Contributes to Weight Management." *Journal of the American College of Nutrition* 23, no. 4 (August 2004): 316–21.

Wolfe, R. "The Underappreciated Role of Muscle in Health and Disease." *American Journal of Clinical Nutrition* 84 (2006): 475–82.

Zizza, C. A., and B. Xu. "Snacking Is Associated with Overall Diet Quality Among Adults." *Journal of the American Dietetic Association* 112, no. 2 (November 11, 2011): 291–96.

CHAPTER 10: TOP PERFORMERS

Howatson, G., et al. "Effect of Tart Cherry Juice (*Prunus cerasus*) on Melatonin Levels and Enhanced Sleep Quality." *European Journal of Nutrition* (October 30, 2011).

Jackman, S. R., et al. "Branched-Chain Amino Acid Ingestion Can Ameliorate Soreness from Eccentric Exercise." *Medicine & Science in Sports and Exercise* 42, no. 5 (2010): 962–70.

Joseph, J. A., B. Shukitt-Hale, and L. M. Willis. "Grape Juice, Berries, and Walnuts Affect Brain Aging and Behavior." *Journal of Nutrition* 139, no. 9 (September 2009): 1813S–17S.

Kim, Y., et al. "Raisins Are a Low to Moderate Glycemic Index Food with a Correspondingly Low Insulin Index." *Nutrition Research* 28, no. 5 (2008): 304–8.

Krikorian, R., et al. "Blueberry Supplementation Improves Memory in Older Adults." *Journal of Agricultural and Food Chemistry* 58, no. 7 (April 14, 2010): 3996–4000.

Kuehl, K. S., et al. "Efficacy of Tart Cherry Juice in Reducing Muscle Pain During Running: A Randomized Controlled Trial." *Journal of the International Society of Sports Nutrition* 7 (2010): 17.

Rondanelli, M., et al. "The Effect of Melatonin, Magnesium, and Zinc on Primary Insomnia in Long-Term Care Facility Residents in Italy: A Double-Blind, Placebo-Controlled Clinical Trial." *Journal of the American Geriatrics Society* 59, no. 1 (January 2011): 82–90.

Shell, W., et al. "A Randomized, Placebo-Controlled Trial of an Amino Acid Preparation on Timing and Quality of Sleep." *American Journal of Therapeutics* 17, no. 2 (March–April 2010): 133–39.

Index